Key Issues in Health

Gavin Mooney is Professor of Health Economics at the University of Aberdeen and Visiting Professor at the Universities of Sydney, Tromsø, Victoria (Wellington) and Århus. He has also written *Economics, Medicine and Health Care* (2nd edition, 1992), to which this book is a companion volume.

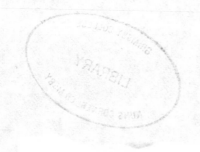

Key Issues in Health Economics

Gavin Mooney

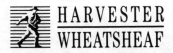

HARVESTER WHEATSHEAF

New York   London   Toronto   Sydney   Tokyo   Singapore

First published 1994 by
Harvester Wheatsheaf
Campus 400, Maylands Avenue
Hemel Hempstead
Hertfordshire, HP2 7EZ
A division of
Simon & Schuster International Group

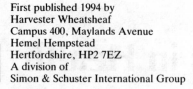

Typeset in 10/12 pt Times
by Keyset Composition, Colchester

Printed and bound in Great Britain by
BPC Wheatons Ltd, Exeter

British Library Cataloguing in Publication Data

A catalogue record for this book is available from
the British Library

ISBN 0-7450-1013-X

2 3 4 5   98 97 96 95 94

To Roy Weir

Contents

Acknowledgements

In preparing this book for publication I have drawn on many experiences gained over the last twenty years or so when I have been a health economist in one guise or another. Over this lengthy period of time, there have been many colleagues and friends to whom I owe a debt for discussing and commenting on my work. In particular I would like to thank Roy Weir, my former boss at the University of Aberdeen, for his encouragement and enthusiasm in establishing the Health Economics Research Unit of which I was Director from 1977 to 1986 and again from 1991 to 1993. I would also like to thank my colleagues there and in the Department of Public Health more generally, especially Elizabeth Russell, Karen Gerard, Mandy Ryan, Ali McGuire, Cam Donaldson, Alastair Gray, Bob and Ann Steele, Ian McAvinchey, Ianthe Fordyce, Brian Yule, Anne Ludbrook and John Cairns.

Beyond that my thanks go to Ivar Sønbø Kristiansen and Jan Abel Olsen of the University of Tromsø; to Jane Hall and Steve Leeder of the University of Sydney; to Uffe Juul Jensen of the University of Århus; to Anita Alban of the Danish Hospital Institute; to Ulrika Enemark of the University of Copenhagen; to Roy Harvey of the Australian Institute of Health and Welfare; to Steve Birch, Amiram Gafni and Greg Stoddart of McMaster University; to Jack Dowie of the Open University; to Tony Culyer, Mike Drummond, Alan Maynard and Alan Williams of the University of York; and to the many students of the Tromsø Distance Learning Course and the Aberdeen Correspondence Course, who have taught me so much in the course of my efforts to teach them.

Finally, my thanks to the many secretaries who have made life so tolerable – no, enjoyable! – for me: Annelise Nielsen, Anne Haastrup, Anne Bews, Linda Hylbech, Kath Latter, Doreen Ellis, Sissel Andersen and especially Isabel Tudhope, but several others besides.

Many organisations have funded me over these years. I am grateful to all of them for their support, but none has responsibility for any errors or idiosyncrasies that emerge in this book.

1

Introduction

Health economics matters. It may be inevitable that I hold this view since I have been working in health economics for twenty years. Trying to use the discipline of economics to encourage more efficiency and equity in health services seems important. Yet I am forced to question this view as health care systems, and especially medical doctors, seem not to embrace some very simple ideas of economics in the way that I would like to see.

Now of course, I can argue that that has to be the fault of all those policy makers and health care professionals who simply want to bury their heads in the sand, hoping that scarcity of resources will go away. But there are other explanations, and I have the feeling that these are more likely to be closer to the truth than the one that I have just presented.

One possibility, of course, is that the economist's message has not been presented in the right way. It is a difficult message very often, and the way that economists use language – and here I mean not so much jargon as simply the English language – has not been helpful. What I hope to do in this book is to allow those who are receptive to the economics message to hear it in a way that I trust will be relatively easy to understand. This I have attempted by selecting a number of issues in health economics where the thinking and techniques of economics seem potentially useful to understanding and analysing better the approaches societies adopt in running and organising their health services.

There are many different perspectives that can be brought to the delivery, financing and consumption of health care but I cannot be shaken from my belief that the contribution of economics is not being taken up to the extent that is desirable. Yet it is being taken up – all health services have to face the strictures of budgetary constraints and of scarce resources. They seem to do so unwillingly, however, and to such a limited and cautious extent that one is almost apologetic about calling oneself a health economist. Economists need to be sensitive (and perhaps have to be oversensitive) to the fact that they cannot expect to receive a warm welcome when bringing the thinking and techniques of economics to bear in an area where pain and suffering are the staple diet of discussion and where there are so many caring people – nurses, doctors, physiotherapists – trying to do their best for their patients. Can it be right to bring the hard-headed logic of economics to issues of health and illness, suffering and death?

Of course it is! If we don't, then pain and suffering will be greater than they need be. The way that health care is distributed will otherwise be less in tune with the wishes of society than it could be. So there is no need for apology. And yet . . .

This book is not intended as an apology, but rather represents an effort on my part to bring this particular economist's thinking to bear on a number of issues in health care where economics has something useful to contribute. It is also my hope that the book will make some of the thinking and ideas of economists – and again, particularly this economist since I make no claims for representing economists more generally – accessible to a health service audience who might otherwise not have the opportunity, even if they were to seek it, to understand economics thinking in health care.

The book is a companion volume to *Economics, Medicine and Health Care*, which is more of an introductory textbook in health economics. However, each book does stand alone. While *Economics, Medicine and Health Care* attempts to adopt a reasonably neutral stance on most of the issues covered there, and to that extent is a textbook in health economics (I know it fails, but I did try!), here I have not even attempted to be neutral. This book is not a review of the evidence, from some sort of objective, scientific stance, on the various topics covered. For it was never my intention to write such a book. I bring my values to this book, and it is perhaps important to the reader that that is made clear in this Introduction. I do not expect readers to agree with all I write. Nor do I think that my views are particularly idiosyncratic. It is my hope that at least some of the ideas expressed here will stimulate the reader to think, and perhaps to think a little differently and from a slightly different perspective, about some of the issues involved in modern health care.

I am encouraged in adopting this stance from experiences with teaching health economics to various non-economist groups in different places. Many health care professionals, and not just formal managers, have a very reasonable, amateur understanding of economics. Very often when I teach I can see nods of 'So that is what that is called in a formal economics sense' or of 'Now I see that more clearly, although I think I understood it anyway from my day-to-day tasks'. There is much that is infuriating about economics and not just for non-economists. I used to get rather upset when I would discover a nurse or doctor (but more often a nurse) who would see through all the smokescreen of theory and concepts, techniques and graphical explanations, and simplify neatly and succinctly, in a few words, some of the heavy structures of economics I had just built into my carefully prepared lecture. Now I see such insights as a bonus. Economics is not some great or wondrous discipline which can work miracles and change low valued water into highly valued wine, or reallocate resources in such a way as to raise the dead. Perhaps, however, it can remove the scales from certain eyes and allow those metaphorically blind to see some of the ways in which health care can be better delivered. If my faith in economics is misplaced, then just put all I have written here down to the arrogance of this economist in his discipline, and put the book back on the shelf. If not, then I exhort you to try to enjoy yourself and certainly do not set out – could there be such a reader? – to agree with all that follows after this.

The selection of topics for inclusion here means that ideally and more accurately this book should have been called 'Some Thought-by-the-author-to-be Key Issues in Health Economics', but that is such a mouthful that I have been happy to go with the less accurate and even more pretentious title of *Key Issues in Health Economics*.

The topics are all ones that I think are important in the context of economics in and of health care, i.e. I think they can be understood better, or acted on better, with an injection of health economics. That range is then restricted further to those which I believe I have some competence to write about. Some are largely policy orientated, such as Chapter 3 dealing with priority setting, others more conceptual (and possibly thought enhancing – I hope so), such as Chapter 6 on agency. I have not attempted to be in any sense comprehensive. I think it is clear that there are many other key issues in health economics, and within topics there is certainly more that could have been said and more evidence presented for and against the cases as I have written them up. The idea, however, is that accessibility should be the dominating concern. There are, of course, opportunities to pursue all the issues in greater detail elsewhere, and I very much hope that this book will stimulate many readers to do just that.

Not only is the book intended to stand alone from *Economics,*

Medicine and Health Care but each chapter is supposed to be able to stand alone, although there is a fair amount of cross-referencing. This means that there is also some repetition in the chapters, especially, as I have discovered in reading through the penultimate draft of the final product, in the recommendations and conclusions at the end of various chapters. As the author, I found this somewhat reassuring! And I trust that the reader will not be bored by this repetition. It is also the case that I think the book is better dipped into than read as a whole. It is for this reason that the strategy of 'stand-alone' chapters was adopted.

A few words about the technical level of the book are appropriate in this Introduction. It is hoped that all the contents will be accessible both to those who have no prior knowledge of economics and to those not very familiar with how the health services work. The language on a few occasions is a little 'economic' in form but most readers who have not encountered economics previously will be able to cope. It will become clear, especially when reading about output measures in Chapter 2 and what it is that people want from their health services in Chapter 11, that economists are very much concerned with the notion of 'utility'. This comes (but not unadulterated!) from the utilitarian school of philosophy with its idea of the greatest good of the greatest number. The reader will have little difficulty in following the discussion of utility and utility functions if he or she remembers the following points. Utility can be equated more or less with satisfaction or happiness or whatever it is that individuals want to maximise. Economists tend to assume that individuals want to maximise their utility and that they do this by maximising whatever utility they get from the 'arguments' in their 'utility functions'. Thus a utility function contains those things or aspects of life ('arguments') that contribute to an individual's utility or, if they are negative, detract from it. These ideas are conventionally wrapped up in what is called 'expected utility theory' (and where the sources of utility are normally constrained to 'consequences' or 'outcomes' and exclude 'processes' or means). The term 'social welfare' is broadly the same phenomenon as utility but at a society level.

Finally in this Introduction, with respect to the style adopted, there may be parts of the text where some health professionals, especially medical doctors, will take offence at some of the ideas presented and some of the criticisms made of the medical profession. It seems often to be the case that the incentives they face push, or at least encourage or allow them to go, in the direction of being inefficient in their behaviour, and consequently that there is a need to see whether and how we can change these incentives. Putting it in these terms – of doctors facing the wrong set of incentives – makes it clear that the 'fault' for the existence of wrong incentives rests not with the medical profession but with the politicians and the policy makers who allow such incentives to continue. I believe that efficiency in health care matters and that it is impossible to have efficient health services without efficient doctors. One of the purposes of this book is to underline that belief, and I hope to do so without offending the profession any more than is absolutely necessary. I am not sure that all doctors who read this book will agree at the end that I have succeeded in this goal. Perhaps those willing to pursue the road to efficiency will be more ready to agree.

The topics

In Chapter 2 I have looked specifically at QALYs *per se*. These again have been seen to be a major advance in measuring health, and I would agree with that assessment. There is, however, a need for caution and that is partly what this chapter is about. In this same chapter, however, I also raise the issue of other outputs of the health care system and especially the question of 'process utility'. Patients and citizens get more from their health service than just health, and some of these other aspects seem best considered as part of the process of health care. The chapter accepts that health outputs are the key but expresses a concern that health ought not to monopolise the thinking of policy makers and analysts on what it is that patients and citizens want from their health service. (I am frequently struck by the fact that when asking friends and colleagues about some involvement they have had with the health care system they talk more about how nice the nurse was or how the doctor failed to communicate well than about the outcome of the treatment. It may be simply that we can all recognise a caring nurse but it is more difficult to pin down what constitutes the actions of a technically competent doctor.)

I have addressed the issue of priority setting in two chapters, one specifically titled priority setting (Chapter 3) and the other dealing with QALY league tables (Chapter 4). At present in health care around the world there is much discussion and policy debate about setting priorities.

Such priority setting has to accept that resources are scarce and that the objective is to try to get as much benefit from available resources as possible, with some consideration at the same time about equity issues. That is about as close to a definition of economics as one can get. Hence it seems that economics ought to be able to make a considerable contribution to the priority-setting debate. The extent to which it does in practice is much more limited than I would expect. This issue, and how economics might tackle the setting of priorities, lies at the heart of these two chapters. The chapter on QALY league tables is in a sense more of a criticism of some of my health economist colleagues than of health care policy makers. QALY league tables may be damaging to the health of a health service, and the message here is that QALY league tables should be seen in their true perspective, accepting that there are both advantages and disadvantages in using them.

With the advent of more and more interest in competition and the use of market forces for the promotion of efficiency in health care, equity in health care is a topic that seems to have been taking something of a back seat in the last few years. Yet equity remains an important goal of most health care systems. Certainly, it seems often to be shrouded in a cloak of confusion and there is too little debate about equity at an operational level. In Chapter 5 on equity, I have tried to spell out some of the main issues as I see them, and certainly have indulged here in pressing my own views. Debate is needed. I hope this chapter will help the reader in any debate on equity with which she or he gets involved.

The notion of the doctor acting as the patient's agent has become a commonplace in health economics and is an issue that has been discussed in the literature for a very long time. However, there is a surprising lack of agreement among health economists as to what the objective of the perfect agent might be. This and other issues related to this rather peculiar aspect of health economics are debated in Chapter 6. In my estimation this is perhaps the area of health policy in which economists have most to contribute after priority setting.

Supplier-induced demand (SID) seems at times one of the corner-stones of health economics and much has been written on the topic. In particular there has been a burgeoning of literature on measuring 'SID'. In Chapter 7, however, I suggest that, as conventionally defined, there is no real possibility of being able to establish whether or not SID exists. I argue that rather than worry about that, health economists should concern themselves more with incentives generally, how doctors behave and how to get them to behave efficiently.

I have always believed that getting the doctor and the patient to act together within the agency relationship to achieve an efficient use of health care resources is the way forward in health policy. It is for this reason that I have put the issue of doctor remuneration and of patient payment together in Chapter 9. I think that this creates an interesting framework for addressing some of the key issues in health care policy.

A closely related issue is that of medical practice variations, which are a blight on the medical profession and on health care more generally. Chapter 8 explores two very different theories which are used to try to explain these variations. Additionally, the chapter looks at what might be done to resolve some of the problems created by these variations.

Chapter 10 on competition is not a review of competition in health generally. That is available from other sources (e.g. Culyer, Maynard and Posnett, 1990; and to some extent also Donaldson and Gerard, 1993). Some of the relevant literature is discussed, but that is *en route* to a debate about the issue of incentives more generally. There is a need to change incentives in many health care systems. Are the incentives of competition the way forward? Are they the best way to go or are other ways preferable? It is these issues that are discussed in Chapter 10.

In an attempt to bring together some thoughts and strands towards the end of the book I have set out a chapter entitled 'What do we want from our health services? What can we expect from out doctors?' This summarises much of what has gone before and suggests that, from a health economics standpoint, we need to pay much more attention to the doctor–patient relationship than health economists have done to date and ask how that relationship can be made to work better. I also raise in Chapter 11 the issue of what not just patients but also citizens want from their health service.

Finally, in Chapter 12 I state briefly why it is that economics is not making the contribution to health services that it might, and what can be done to improve the position. I have drawn here on some work that has been done in Australia, Denmark and the United Kingdom on understanding from policy makers what the problems are in using economics to assist them. I think there is scope for optimism here but that may be not so much a considered, objective assessment as a reflection of the fact that this book is written by an optimist and one who happens to be a health economist!

References

Culyer, A. J., Maynard, A. and Posnett, J. (1990) *Competition in Health Care, Reforming the NHS*. Macmillan, London.
Donaldson, C. and Gerard, K. (1993) *Economics of Health Care Financing*. Macmillan, London.

2
Health care outputs – and processes

Introduction

When health care outputs are discussed it is very often assumed that the only output is health. Indeed, in recent years a research industry has grown up which tries to measure health. What seems very often to be forgotten is that while it is reasonable to assume that the objective of health care will be dominated by the pursuit of health, there are other objectives, and certainly other effects, that health services have which have an impact on how individuals *qua* individuals and as a society feel. What effects other than health changes make people feel better or make them feel worse? What aspects of health services affect what economists call the 'utility' of individuals and 'social welfare' more generally (see p. 4 in Chapter 1 on utility)?

I shall examine in this chapter a number of issues related to both health status measurement and other changes likely to occur in utility for individuals who consume health care, and in two instances the impact on that utility of changes which affect individuals who do not have access to health care. These take the form of 'regret' for those who, in a sense, make a wrong choice and then regret it; and deprivation, which arises when, for example, an individual is debarred from a service or is ineligible for it but knows that it exists for others.

The arguments I want to consider are the following. First, information: how does this fit into the utility function? Is information solely about reducing uncertainty, or does it have value in itself? And in so far as it does have value, is this only in terms of its impact on health and do we need any additional measure here, or will QALYs (quality adjusted life years), or perhaps some other measure of health, adequately embrace the value of information through health? More specifically, how does information sit together with reassurance and anxiety?

Second is the issue of decision making *per se*. As discussed at greater length in Chapter 6 on agency, there is the possibility at least that individual consumers of health care get utility from the fact that there is an agent to help them to make better and more informed decisions than would otherwise be the case. It is assumed that this influence goes beyond that of any impact on health or information. The individual values the possibility of being able to pass difficult decisions to the agent and so avoid the problems of having to make the decisions herself.

Third and related, but not quite the same point, even if there is an overlap, there is the question of autonomy and having the right to make one's decisions and having that right respected. The concept of autonomy is important in medical decision making but it is one that economists have apparently not given much consideration to and indeed seem sometimes to equate (I would submit wrongly) with consumer sovereignty.

Fourth, there are potentially relevant variables related to waiting for treatment, which may have a bearing on the issue of deprivation but which would seem to cover other aspects as well.

Finally, I think there are aspects of health care consumption that can be described as process variables, which may be utility- or disutility-bearing for consumers. Here I am thinking of circumstances surrounding being treated. These may stretch from issues of the way in which a GP's receptionist deals with patients, to the effects of preparing for a contrast X-ray, through the discomfort of a rectal examination, to aspects of embarrassment in having a breast screening examination. Some of these are sometimes considered under the heading 'patient satisfaction', which seems primarily concerned with what might be described as non-health or non-clinical variables. But it is precisely these variables that seem not to be considered by economists when looking at the output of the health care system.

QALYs

Quality Adjusted Life Years (QALYs) have become very popular in health economics in recent years and indeed beyond health economics. They are primarily associated with George Torrance in Canada and Alan Williams in the United Kingdom. They have been devised as a mechanism to measure health with a view to getting a useful, quantified measure of the output of individual programmes in health care. This allows, from an economic point of view, estimates to be made of the relative efficiency of different procedures in tackling the same problem or the allocative efficiency questions of where to invest more in the development of the health care system. In other words, on this latter front they are claimed to be helpful in deciding where the 'best buys' are likely to be for new investment in health care (see, for example, Torrance, 1986; Williams, 1985).

Precisely what are QALYs? Despite their popularity there is less than agreement among economists as to what they are. It is helpful, however, to consider this question by looking at how QALYs are measured.

There are principally three ways of measuring QALYs, each of which is concerned to bring together in a single measuring scale which is perhaps best described as 'health state utilities', both mortality and morbidity aspects of health. These respectively are sometimes called the quantity aspects and the quality aspects, although these terms are somewhat misleading, as it is difficult to envisage quantity of life which has no quality aspects to it. (Indeed when it comes to interpersonal comparisons, this separation of quantity from quality tends to conceal potential differences, at least some of which may be important in practice.)

Let us take the 'time trade-off' method of estimating QALYs. This involves a series of questions put to respondents along the lines of 'Would you prefer 10 years in state X or 20 years in state Y?' where state Y is a worse state of health than state X. Now if state X is perfect health and the respondent is indifferent between the two choices when there is an equivalence when the length of time in state Y is 15 years, then state Y is being 'valued' at two-thirds of perfect health and is therefore weighted as 0.67. It is then considered that, if an individual is in this state of health for 10 years, the number of QALYs this represents is 6.7, and further that if the individual can be moved from that state to perfect health for the 10-year period, then the QALYs gained by this amount to 3.3, i.e. $10 \times 1 - 10 \times 0.67$.

When we move to consider this sort of situation across a range or group of people, the QALY weight will normally be taken as some weighted average of the population's values, so that we end up with a situation whereby everyone who has 10 years to live and who experiences this gain in utility is attributed with a gain of 3.3 QALYs if the average for the group is 3.3. Further, if there are 100 individuals in the group, the total gain is 330 QALYs and this gain is the same as if 33 people had an extended life of 10 years in perfect health, i.e. $33 \times 10 \times 1$.

A number of issues arise from this. First, there is no allowance for different preferences with respect to health *per se* across different individuals. Everyone who has an extension of life of 10 years in perfect health is assumed to have the same utility gain. That is, all years in perfect health are assumed to be equally valuable no matter who gets them and no matter how they are distributed. Even though some individuals may value health more highly than others, this is not taken into account in the way that QALYs are calculated and used.

Second, departures from perfect health are valued equally, no matter the individual involved and no matter that some individuals may value such losses in health status more than others. The loss of use of a leg or arm is valued the same whether the individuals concerned are concert pianists, fast bowlers or health economists. Thus again, there is no allowance for strengths of preferences varying among different individuals with respect to their disutility associated with loss in health status.

Third, there is no allowance for 'diminishing marginal utility of health'. As an individual receives more and more health gains, in reality the benefit from each additional health gain is likely to diminish. QALYs do not normally allow for this phenomenon. This assumption, that there is no diminishing marginal utility of health, also means that the gains in health are unaffected by the level of health status before any health gain occurs. A QALY is a QALY is a QALY no matter who gets it or how many that person already has, or how many he or she is gaining with any particular change in health care.

Fourth, there is no independence of health states across different time periods. While there may be an allowance for discounting because of time (i.e. that health improvements occurring further into the future, *ceteris paribus*, are valued less highly in the present than those occurring in the nearer future) there is an assumption that a quality adjustment applies irrespective of the length of time that the health state exists. Thus to be unable to get out and about without help for 10 years is valued at 10 times what being in that state is for 1 year. Similarly, being in a certain state for 2 seconds – say, extreme pain – is valued at one-eighteen-hundredth of what it would be in being in that state for 1 hour. (For more discussion of discounting QALYs see, for example, Olsen, 1993.)

These issues are all somewhat problematical. However, the extent to which they undermine QALYs as measures of health is largely an empirical question. Do they seriously distort what it is that QALYs claim to represent or that they are practically useful in representing? (These are clearly not the same thing!)

Two conclusions emerge from this discussion. First, health economists have to be careful in how they represent QALYs and indicate clearly what their strengths and weaknesses are. Second, since the extent of difficulties associated with these issues is largely an empirical question, research is needed to measure the influence of these problems in different circumstances.

One of the issues that arises is what we are to use as a 'golden standard' when looking at QALYs. The answer is that there probably is no 'golden standard' even if 'healthy years equivalent' are a better measure in at least one respect. (For more detailed assessments of 'HYEs', see Mehrez and Gafni, 1989; and Culyer and Wagstaff, 1992.) HYEs avoid the assumption of the independence of each year's health status on other years and that the quality of life in one period may have an influence on the quality of life in another. While this does seem to be a potentially major advantage over QALYs, the disadvantage is that it means that developing and working with HYEs is more difficult than with QALYs.

Are QALYs a measure of utility, this satisfaction index that economists want to use? They are utility-*based* in the sense that they do contain elements of preferences of individuals with respect to different states of the world, and they do allow aggregation of these preferences for individuals and across individuals, subject to the constraints and problems outlined above (especially with respect to interpersonal comparisons of utility and aggregation more generally). They do not, however, allow variations in preferences for the same health state among different individuals. Further, they are constrained within health and tell us nothing about the relationship between preferences for health and preferences for any other state of the world. To that extent they cannot legitimately be called utility measures which have more general applicability, but only preferences within the context of health and different states of the health world. They are thus better called 'health state utilities' (Torrance, 1986).

Now that is a useful thing to be able to do, so I need to be careful that I do not appear to overstate my concerns about QALYs. But as I highlight in Chapter 4, when considering the issue of QALY league tables, there are limitations on QALYs in certain circumstances which have perhaps not been adequately spelt out. They cannot be used to make judgements about the amount of health care *in toto* that 'should' be supplied to a community. In principle it is possible to arrive at a figure representing the marginal cost per QALY across all programmes which, within a given budget, indicates the optimal way of allocating resources within the budget, assuming (1) that QALYs measure what we want them to measure, and (2) that there is nothing else that influences (or should influence) decision makers in what they want to achieve than the maximisation of QALYs within that budget. But the key point here is that this is viable as a decision rule *only within a given budget*.

It has been suggested that there is some cut-off point which can be used to decide on allocations of monies both to and within health care. QALYs do not help with the first issue but they can in principle help with the second once a particular budget is set. But getting to that point also requires that all procedures and programmes are examined through cost–utility studies. We are a long way from that (as Gerard (1992) has indicated), but there are certainly advantages in keeping that goal in mind when setting health care priorities.

If we do want to go further and consider the question of how much to spend on health care as compared with other ways of using society's resources, then cost–utility analysis has to be replaced with cost–benefit analysis. This latter technique, of course, also has the advantage of including legitimately more types of benefit than just health and more types of cost than just health service costs.

Beyond these issues there are the questions of how best to measure QALYs, who is to be involved in the measuring and what the best way to use QALYs is. (I suppose to what extent their use should be constrained to particular issues might be a better way to phrase this concern.) These issues are currently not resolved in the literature. With respect to which method to use for measuring QALYs there are three possibilities: (1) the analogue scale; (2) the time trade-off method; and (3) the standard gamble. The first of these normally operates on the basis that a line running from 1 to 0 represents the distance between two health states – say, perfect health and death respectively – and respondents are asked to place some intermediate health state, e.g. a broken leg, on the line. If the point were, say, 0.9, then being in the state of health 'broken leg' would be considered by the respondent to be 90 per cent as good as perfect health, or to involve 10 per cent loss of health.

Time trade-off (which was used as an example above) means just that, and involves giving respondents a choice between two health states which are different and in which they are expected to spend different lengths of time. Thus the choice might be between perfect health for 10 years or living with continual pain for 12 years or 15 years or 20 years. The length of life chosen by the individual for the period in continual pain allows a calculation of the value of the state of health 'continual pain' as compared with perfect health. If the individual chooses 20 years, then this means that continual pain is valued at just 50 per cent of being in perfect health.

With the standard gamble the choices involved are probabilistic: would an individual prefer the certainty of health state X (which is less than perfect) for 10 years followed by death, or some probability of perfect health for 10 years followed by death and 1– that probability of immediate death. When the individual is indifferent with a probability of p, then that p represents the value of state X when perfect health equals 1.

There has been considerable debate in the literature about which is the best method. That is necessary as it does seem to be the case that the methods produce different results and are not equally easy for respondents to comprehend. They may actually be measuring different things. For example, the analogue scale does not involve any concept of choice while the other two do, and it may be that that is one reason at least why the analogue scale gives different results. Again, the probabilistic approach of the standard gamble may allow some idea of attitude to risk to be incorporated. But even this is disputed in the literature to some extent, and I believe legitimately so. There seems little consensus, and for the present that is all that I want to establish. However, it is worth noting that the methods probably do measure different things. Perhaps the differences between the methods are legitimate and the choice is one of what best relates to the problems to hand.

On the question of who is to do the valuing, most commentators seem to think that 'community values' should be the basis for QALYs. However, this depends to some extent on how the results are to be used. Where we are concerned only with how best to screen for breast cancer, then using women's values or the values of women at risk would seem to be appropriate. Where, however, we are concerned to compare the allocative efficiency issue of breast cancer screening versus neonatal intensive care, then community values would seem better.

There is, however, the question of whether the analysts should answer the question: whose values? My view would be that the community should determine this as well as the health state utility values. How can this be achieved? It would be possible at the same time as obtaining QALY values to ask about the weights to be given to different individuals' values or different groups' values in the process. Thus we could ask respondents: 'If these values are to be used in decisions about which method of breast screening to adopt, what weight do you think should be attached to the values of the following groups in society?' (and there we might list such groups as: women; women with breast cancer; women at risk of breast cancer; men; men with female partners; etc.). Again, we might ask this question but indicate that the values were to be used to address the relative priorities to be given to breast cancer screening, neonatal intensive care and geriatric respite care for the relatives of the elderly.

There will be other ways of deciding how the QALY values should be established. However, there does seem merit in trying to use community preferences when deciding whose values to use and to allow for the fact that the answer to that question may vary depending on how the QALYs are to be used, i.e. what problem they are being used for.

Which questions should they be used to answer? There seems little doubt that, faced with questions of the relative effectiveness of alternative treatments for the same health condition, using QALYs will have considerable advantage over many and possibly all single-dimension measures, such as mortality or survival which have been commonly used in the past in clinical trials. And they are likely to be preferred in those circumstances over intermediate measures, such as cases treated or the extent of lowering cholesterol levels or blood pressure, etc. They are then likely to be useful at the level of operational efficiency as well as when comparing different ways of treating a particular condition in terms of costs per QALY. Where there has to be more doubt about their value is in allocative efficiency and where, even in questions of effectiveness or operational efficiency, there are important influences not covered by health and where there may be major differences in resource use outside the health care system, e.g. when there are major differences in terms of patients' inputs of time.

Also, when the answers to questions are likely to be influenced markedly by equity considerations, QALYs may be deficient in that it is clear that, in so far as they can deal with equity, it can only be if such equity is seen in terms of equality of health. If, as discussed in the chapter on equity (see Chapter 5), there are other considerations in the dimension of equity which are considered relevant, such as use or access, QALYs cannot deal adequately with these.

Other outcomes and process issues

As indicated in the Introduction, much of the literature on outcomes in health care is concerned solely with health, on the grounds either that that is the only outcome of the health care system or that health is the only one that is deemed relevant when examining health care policies from the standpoint of economic appraisal. In what follows I speculate about other possible arguments that may arise in patients' and citizens' utility functions; in other words, what other health care factors may affect individuals' utilities.

Equity of access

Elsewhere (Mooney and Olsen, 1991) I have suggested that QALYs may not be enough, in so far as they do not consider equity, especially in the Margolis (1982) context of allowing a concern for 'doing our fair share'. The Margolis model assumes that each individual has two utility functions, one concerned with a 'standard' neoclassical 'goods' utility function, the other with the utility derived from what Margolis calls 'participation utility'. Margolis assumes that individuals are prepared to contribute to 'group utility' (where each individual is a member of the group and as likely to obtain utility from the use of group resources as any other member of the group). They derive utility from the act of participating.

Here is a means of incorporating equity in health care within the individual's utility function. Individuals get utility from providing services which are then available to all. (All have access to them.) This utility arises from the act of provision – 'doing our fair share' – rather than from the utility that the individuals in the group obtain from their use of these resources. This is particularly relevant when equity is so often defined in terms of access rather than of health care use or of health. The utility arises from the 'participation' in the providing rather than in the use or in the health gains arising from such use. In more normal terminology, it arises through individuals contributing so that everyone has equal access to health care services.

One of the operational disadvantages of moving the equity target away from health *per se* is that it means that there is an argument in the utility function which concerns not health but access to health care.

One interesting recent piece of research in this field comes from Australia. Hall (1993) investigated the change in health status over time which followed in the wake of the introduction of Medicare in Australia in 1984. She examined health status changes, first among those who had previously not had access to insured care and who under Medicare were so insured (and therefore whose access had been improved by the introduction of this universal coverage); and second among those who were covered both before and after the introduction of Medicare. She found no evidence to suggest that the introduction of Medicare had led to any increase in the health of previously uninsured.

This raises the interesting question of whether this policy of universal access in Australia has 'failed'. Clearly, it is difficult to set up an ideal measure of health status to allow such changes to be monitored accurately and validly. While there is no intended criticism of Hall's efforts in this respect, none the less there are clear problems in attempting such an exercise. However, let us assume that the lack of significant change in Hall's study accurately reflects what happened to the health of the previously uninsured. Should the Commonwealth Government of Australia abandon Medicare? Additional resources have been expended in health care on the basis of a concern for equity. Yet if that equity concern is to be viewed in terms solely of health, Medicare appears not to have improved the position. Are the people of Australia only concerned for the health of the population because, if so, Medicare should presumably be abandoned. But if the people of Australia gain utility from 'Margolis participation' (as described above) and thereby in this context through paying the Medicare levy on income, there might be sufficient utility gains from this to justify Medicare, even if the health status of the poor has not been improved.

It is not my intention to be normative here by implying that people 'ought' to get utility from 'participation', or 'ought' to get utility through improving equality of access. My point rather is to suggest that there may be an argument present in individuals' utility functions that goes beyond health. This would be seen in terms of contributing to the provision of health care to allow more equal access (even if the use did not increase or the health status improve).

Information

In the context of the evaluation of a prenatal diagnostic test for autosomal polycystic kidney disease (APKD), I have attempted, with Mette Lange, to show – and indeed would suggest that we have shown – that the individuals at risk whom we surveyed indicated a willingness to pay (quite substantial amounts) for information *per se* (Mooney and Lange, 1993).

Most at-risk individuals were willing to pay to have a test during pregnancy to show whether or not the affected gene was present in the foetus. For at-risk individuals there is a 50 per cent chance that a foetus will be affected. If such an affected gene is present this will mean that the individual will suffer from polycystic kidney disease. This will normally be symptomless until the age of about 40 or 50. Thereafter it is likely to lead to end-stage renal disease, requiring either a kidney transplant or renal dialysis. Before the onset of end-stage renal disease there is little that can be done to treat or slow the progression of the disease. Overall, therefore, the disease is very different from, say, Down's syndrome and essentially means a shortening of life expectation by perhaps 10 years with relatively few morbidity effects.

Interestingly in the context of the utility of information, approximately half of our (admittedly small) sample were prepared to pay for the test without proceeding to choose to abort if the foetus were shown to be affected. Certainly it could be that this information was seen as relevant to the management of the birth and the impact on the woman of the discovery of the problem after birth. However, while this might seem a rational explanation if we were dealing with Down's, given the nature of APKD this seems unlikely. We argue that this represents utility in information *per se*. (I appreciate that most of the literature on information in economics does not allow for the possibility of utility in information *per se* but rather treats it as a reduction in uncertainty or in altering the expected utility of future consumption of some other good about which the information is concerned. I think in this case, though, that this is utility in information *per se*.)

More generally, together with others, I have been looking recently at the nature of the benefits that flow from a breast cancer screening programme (Lange *et al.*, 1991). Here we have identified six groups of women who are affected by the existence or creation of such a screening programme. For those who are screened there are potential health effects for the true positives, for the false positives and for those screened false negative. But it can be argued that there are also information effects for all these groups and additionally for the true negatives. (I would include reassurance here as being a function of information and not as a separate argument in the woman's utility function. I discuss the other two of the six groups on p. 21.

That information is a relevant argument in women's utility functions in such instances seems quite clear. Again there is a study by Berwick and Weinstein (1985) which appears to show that there is an argument in pregnant women's utility functions that is concerned with information – in this case in the context of ultrasound in normal pregnancy.

One interesting aspect of these examples is that they are restricted to screening. If there is an information argument in individuals' utility functions, it is easy to argue that it is likely to have greater weight in the context of screening than in, say, treatment programmes. There is less evidence to date that patients in treatment regimes obtain utility (or disutility) from information. However, I would argue that while the weight attached to information may be less in treatment programmes, none the less it is likely to be present. In other words, and contrary to what is normally assumed in expected utility theory and in the QALY literature, information is likely to be present in the patient's utility function. More empirical evidence, however, is needed.

Autonomy and decision making

Yet another argument in the patient's utility function relates to the issue of autonomy. Here I use the word differently from the meaning implied in consumer sovereignty. With consumer sovereignty, economists tend to go beyond the basic idea that individuals are the best judge of their own welfare, and use consumer sovereignty to suggest that this applies to consumption choices. In other words, the fact of consumer sovereignty leads on to the idea that it is the individual's values that are to be used in consumption choices and that it is the consumer who is to make the consumption choices. Autonomy (which interestingly does not appear in my dictionary of economics) is defined as being a wider concept, which gives the individual the right not only to make the consumption choices but also the right not to make the consumption choices. This important distinction allows choice (and/or ability to pass choice to an agent) to enter as an argument in the consumer's utility function. Because of its reliance on consumer sovereignty, expected utility theory does not allow for choice as an argument in the utility function. (We have here a 'process' variable as I have discussed with others elsewhere; see McGuire *et al.*, 1988.)

It is unfortunate that in the medical literature the word autonomy has several meanings and that in the wake of the move towards 'consumerism' in health care, little thought seems to be given to whether the patient wants to exercise choice. For example, in the reforms of the NHS there is an inbuilt assumption that 'consumption choice' is a 'good thing'. It is not at all clear this is necessarily the case (nor that UK consumers have been asked!). In this context, there seems to be a strong argument for economists to analyse the medical literature on informed consent which, rather crudely, seems very often to be about doctor utility rather than patient utility. In other words, informed consent allows the doctor to shed some of her risk bearing on to the patient with the result that the patient may suffer disutility not only from this increased risk bearing but also from the receipt of the information *per se*. Here ignorance on the part of the patient may be bliss and under my proposed definition of autonomy would be respected. However, where autonomy moves in the direction of assuming that there must be utility in exercising informed choice, whatever the outcome and whatever the utility the patient derives from such choosing, then there is a departure from the way in which I am suggesting the concept of autonomy is used in the patient's utility function.

There are, in fact, different views of autonomy even in the philosophy literature. The idea that the patient should decide because it is good for her and as such is a defence against paternalism (which is seen as being 'bad') is what is normally defined as 'deontological autonomy'. It embodies the normative concept that patients 'should' make their own decisions. The way in which I have set out autonomy above is closer to the notion of 'relativistic autonomy'. (For more discussion, see Jensen and Mooney, 1990.)

Process

Most of the economics literature on the topic of health care outputs is based on expected utility theory. As mentioned in the section above on autonomy and decision making, some possible effects that may have an impact on individuals' utility, such as choice *per se*, may be excluded under this theory. This theory is 'consequentialist' in the sense that it assumes that the only aspects of health care that have an impact on utility are outcomes and not processes – ends, in other words, and not means.

In practice, it can sometimes be quite difficult to sort out what is an outcome and what is a process. Dowie (1993), for example, argues that all relevant effects (or arguments in the utility function) can be accommodated under the notion of outcome utility and that it is not necessary to create some new phenomenon of 'process utility' to cover such matters as choice, respect, dignity, being treated kindly by the hospital staff, etc. He does not dispute the potential relevance of these aspects of process to the utility of patients. Dowie's position can be summed up in what he calls both the title and the abstract of his paper: 'Process utility' can seriously damage your health service evaluation but the generic measure of benefit should include 'service outcomes'. He includes in his list of attributes relevant to health service economic evaluation various 'outcomes' which seem to me more like 'processes': for example, 'cared for/dignity state'; and 'autonomy/self-determination state'.

Here I do not want to debate whether or not it is necessary to create some new concept of process utility. What Dowie and I do agree on is that there is a need to widen research into health care outputs to include not just health and not just conventionally described outcomes. There are various processes that patients (and perhaps also citizens – see the discussion above on equity of access) undergo that may well be utility bearing and which as such ought to be included in looking at the utility of health care services.

Deprivation

There is a literature in economics which considers various facets of utility beyond that of the conventional expected utility theory. I do not intend to summarise that literature here, but none the less draw on it. In essence what I want to suggest is that there may well be legitimate reasons why doctors and others will want to reject QALYs when such QALYs are based solely on expected utility theory, as they tend to be in their current incarnation.

Let me look briefly at some of the arguments (for a review, see Loomes and McKenzie, 1989; and Mooney and Olsen, 1991). First, QALYs normally assume that $U(H1 - H2) = U(H1) - U(H2)$. In other words QALYs, being expected utility theory-based, assume that what is utility bearing is states of the world and that the difference in utility in moving from state H1 to state H2 is the same as the numerical difference between the utility in state H1 and the utility in state H2. That seems questionable.

There is some evidence to support the view that the utility of a health state is not independent of the recent health state of the respondent, and it seems very likely would be a function of the current health state of the respondent. People appear to adjust to health states in the sense that the expected and realised utility may well vary as a result of some form of learning and/or coping process (see, for example, Nord, 1992). Prospect theory can take this into account. There would seem to be much to be said for economists trying to work more with the sort of model that Kahneman and Tversky (1979) have developed under prospect theory. Yet I know of no current work which is building QALYs specifically on the basis of prospect theory.

Here I want to look at regret theory (see for example, Loomes and Sugden, 1982). Let me return to the breast cancer screening example raised above (Lange *et al.*, 1991). When a breast screening opportunity arises, women who are deemed eligible can choose whether or not to be screened. Regret would arise if a woman chose not to be screened and then subsequently discovered that she had a breast cancer that could have been detected at an earlier stage if she had chosen to be screened. Here, one of the preconditions for the existence of regret is choice. The eligible woman made a personal choice not to be screened. She is worse off after choosing not to be screened than if the screening programme had not existed.

In fact, in the context of screening I have identified with others (Lange *et al.*, 1991) six groups of women whose utility is potentially affected by access to a screening programme. We have discussed earlier four of these groups – the true and false positives, and the true and false negatives, i.e. the women screened. But there are two other groups of women whose utility may be affected by the existence of a screening programme.

First, there are those women who, although eligible for screening,

choose not to be screened and then suffer regret as a result of choosing not to take up the offer. Second are those women who are not eligible, and it is here that 'deprivation disutility' comes into play. It may be that such a screening programme is restricted to women over 50 and the under-fifties feel deprived. Or, in the context of screening for Down's syndrome, a 34-year-old woman is not eligible because the cut-off point is 35 and only older women can be screened. Younger women, whatever the outcome of their pregnancy, may feel 'deprived' and, even when their risk of giving birth to a Down's baby is unchanged, may suffer greater disutility than would be the case if the test for Down's did not exist at all. Of course, this assumes that the women know of the existence of the test and of their exclusion from it. It is important to note that, as compared with regret, deprivation does not involve choice on the part of the patient. Indeed, it is a precondition for the existence of deprivation disutility that the patient is deprived of choosing to have the service concerned.

This concept may be relevant in a number of areas of health care. Here the decision context is something that economists appear not to take sufficient account of when discussing patients' utility functions, and which the QALY literature ignores completely. Yet as Evans and Wolfson (1980) note: 'it is easier to bear inevitable disease or death than to learn that remedy is possible but one's personal resources, private insurance coverage or public programme will not support it.'

For example, if a new technology is introduced, before it is widely disseminated it is likely that it will be restricted to a number of patients, perhaps in a particular geographical area. In this case, those who live elsewhere may suffer 'deprivation disutility' and be worse off than if the technology had never been introduced. (All of this assumes, of course, that these 'deprived' patients know of the existence of the technology.)

It follows that the existence of such disutility can be used as part of the reasoning for ensuring that access to this new technology is extended to all those potentially 'eligible', although this may not totally overcome the presence of deprivation disutility if the criterion for eligibility is based solely on some cost per QALY type of calculations. Again, much depends on the 'decision environment'.

'Deprivation disutility' may also be relevant to certain forms of analysis of waiting lists. Assume, for example, that I am on a waiting list when others are getting access to health care (for example, where a private market exists alongside a public one and the private market affords faster access to hospital care). Having to wait has its disutility; but having to wait knowing that others, who are similarly placed, do not may create another form of deprivation.

Many hold the view that if a particular form of treatment exists, then all who might benefit from it should have access to it. Birk (1991), for example, found that of a sample of GP patients, over 90 per cent agreed or strongly agreed with the statement: 'If the public authorities sought to offer a test – for detecting cystic fibrosis – to anyone, then everyone in Denmark who wants it should have access to it.' Clearly, such a view runs counter to the cost per QALY league table method of sorting out priorities. If applied, it would mean that, if societies had a particularly strong preference for such a criterion, then the question of which services to introduce and when would need to take more account of the eligibility criterion than is currently the case. It is in a sense a strong equity principle, yet it is not based on the same Margolis consideration for equity through participation discussed earlier in this chapter (Margolis, 1982). Indeed, it is a much more 'selfishly' based form of utility. It is the feeling on the part of an individual suffering from some problem that, since someone else is suffering from the same problem and is eligible for a particular form of treatment, then so should that individual. It is not that the first individual envies the second. It is perfectly possible that the concept of a 'caring external-ity', i.e. individuals care about others in some way or other, may operate here alongside that of deprivation disutility.

Conclusions

There are three conclusions that I would want readers to draw from this series of thoughts about the patient's utility function. First, as economists we need to do more work on attempting to find out rather than just assuming that we (along with doctors) already know what is in the patient's utility function. Second, we need to consider more carefully the decision environment in which any measures of output are to be used in economic evaluations. Both the arguments in the utility function and the weights attached to them may well be decision specific. And third, we need to measure what we should measure rather than measure and model something else because it is more readily measured and modelled. That is a fate that has befallen much of the work in equity. It seems important that we do not fall into the same trap when we attempt to measure the outputs of the health care system.

References

Berwick, D. M. and Weinstein, M. C. (1985) What do patients value? Willingness to pay for ultrasound in pregnancy. *Medical Care*, **23**, 881–93.

Birk, H. O. (1991) Udledning af pyttefunktionen med hensyn til sundhedsydelser, Stor opgave (Development of a utility function for health services). Master's dissertation, Department of Economics, University of Copenhagen, Copenhagen.

Culyer, A. J. and Wagstaff, A. (1992) QALYs versus HYEs: a theoretical exposition. Discussion paper 99, Centre for Health Economics, University of York, York.

Dowie, J. (1993) 'Process utility' can seriously damage your health service evaluation but the generic measure of benefit should include 'service outcomes'. Paper presented to the Health Economists' Study Group meeting, July 1993, Glasgow.

Evans, R. G. and Wolfson, A. D. (1980) Faith, hope and charity: health care in the utility function. Discussion paper, Department of Economics, University of British Columbia, Vancouver.

Gerard, K. (1992) Cost utility in practice: a policy maker's guide to the state of the art. *Health Policy*, **21**, 249–79.

Hall, J. (1993) Equity in Health Care, PhD thesis, Department of Public Health, University of Sydney, Sydney.

Jensen, U. J. and Mooney, G. (1990) *Changing Values in Medical and Health Care Decision Making*. Wiley, London.

Kahneman, D. and Tversky, A. (1979) Prospect theory: an analysis of decision making under risk. *Econometrica*, **47**, 2, 263–91.

Lange, M., Gerard, K., Turnbull, D. and Mooney, G. (1991) Economic evaluation of mammography screening: information reassurance and anxiety. CHERE monograph, Department of Community Medicine, University of Sydney, Sydney.

Loomes, G. and McKenzie, L. (1989) The scope and limitations of QALY measures. *Social Science and Medicine*, **28**, 299–308.

Loomes, G. and Sugden, R. (1982) Regret theory; an alternative theory of rational choice under uncertainty. *Economic Journal*, **92**, 805–24.

Margolis, H. (1982) *Selfishness, Altruism and Rationality*. Cambridge University Press, Cambridge.

McGuire, A. J., Henderson, J. B. and Mooney, G. H. (1988) *The Economics of Health Care*. Routledge and Kegan Paul, London.

Mehrez, A. and Gafni, A. (1989) Quality adjusted life years, utility theory and healthy-year equivalents. *Medical Decision Making*, **9**, 142–9.

Mooney, G. and Lange, M. (1993) Ante-natal screening: what constitutes benefit? *Social Science and Medicine*, **37**, 7, 873–8.

Mooney, G. and Olsen, J. A. (1991) QALYs: what next? In: A. J. McGuire, P. Fenn and K. Mayhew, *Providing Health Care: The Economics of Alternative Systems of Finance and Delivery*. Oxford University Press, Oxford.

Nord, E. (1992) Methods for quality adjustment for life years. *Social Science and Medicine*, **34**, 5, 559–69.

Olsen, J. A. (1993) On what basis should health be discounted? *Journal of Health Economics*, **12**, 39–53.

Torrance, G. W. (1986) Measurement of health state utilities for economic appraisal. *Journal of Health Economics*, **5**, 1–30.

Williams, A. (1985) Economics of coronary artery bypass grafting. *British Medical Journal*, 326–9.

3

Priority setting in health care

Introduction

There is a sense in which priority setting is what economics is all about. Economics is the science or the art of choice. Limited resources are to be allocated in such a way as to maximise benefits and at the same time ensure that health care is allocated in a way that is fair in the eyes of the society served.

This chapter makes two key points. First, there is a lack of agreement in policy circles as to how best to set priorities in health care. Second, if economics cannot make a contribution to the process of priority setting, it is hard to see to which other aspects of health care economists can contribute. This has to be the key target for economic analysis in health care.

This chapter does three things. First, it sets out how economic analysis can be used to help to set priorities in health care. Second, it outlines various ways of examining priorities which are being used or have been used in health care, identifying at the same time some of the problems from an economic perspective in these approaches. Third, it indicates what might be done to try to get the economic approach used more often in priority setting in health care.

While writing this chapter I was aware of the frustrations I feel that economics seems not to have been accepted more in the field of priority setting. The merits of the economic approach to priority setting seem so obvious to me. Using economic analysis in an ideal fashion can be difficult, given in particular the demands on measuring techniques especially of the benefits of health care, which are still at best developing. There are also data deficiencies in all health care systems in the sense that on both the costs and the benefits side the information does not exist in the form, detail and precision that we would want.

Yet a lot of these measurement and data problems are there *whatever* methods are used to address priorities; and frequently the methods adopted are deficient. We cannot set rational priorities in health care without knowing about the costs and benefits of different patterns of intervention. That is simply impossible. So it is not that the approaches of economics to priority setting create these problems. They exist. In so far as other approaches sidestep these problems they cannot be genuinely useful methods of priority setting in getting us further down the road to more efficient and equitable health services.

This issue seems important. Most of the criticisms that I hear of the economic approach to priority setting seem to centre largely on the practical problems of implementing the approach. They do not, as far as I interpret them, say that the economic approach is wrong, or that it will fail to promote efficiency, or that efficiency and equity are inappropriate objectives of health care. The concerns are almost exclusively with the data demands and the demands on measuring techniques that the economic approach makes. True – but true of all approaches to health care priority setting that will further greater efficiency and equity.

In the opening chapter to this book I tried to emphasise that economics is first and foremost about a way of thinking about resource allocation. In priority setting this is especially true. The key message of this chapter is that unless the thinking underlying priority setting is 'right' – and yes, there is scope for debate about what that means – then there is no possibility except by luck of getting priorities set in such a way that they will further the objectives of health care. It may well be the case – I would say *will* be the case – in the foreseeable future that economic analysis in priority setting will not be implemented in any ideal fashion. However, an inadequate data and measuring set supporting the right thinking is more likely to get us to an approximation of where we want to be than will better data and better measuring techniques where the thinking is wrong.

I debate this issue in some detail in Chapter 12 and the reader might like to glance at certain aspects of that chapter when reading this chapter. But this chapter does stand alone without reference to Chapter 12.

Priority setting using an explicit economics approach

The essence of priority setting from an economics perspective starts from the assumption that resources are scarce. This raises two considerations. First, the concept of opportunity cost is to the fore; and second, the idea of meeting total need is simply not possible and indeed not worthy of contemplation. The starting point is therefore resources.

This means getting an idea of how resources are currently being used and this is best done through programme budgeting. Thereafter, the question to be addressed is how best any changes in resources can be made, be it through some redeployment of existing resources, reductions in existing resources or increases in existing resources. This is the process normally referred to as 'marginal analysis'. It is simple and involves considering whether a shift of resources of, say, Z from programme, project or procedure A to programme, project or procedure B will result in an increase in total benefits from the resources available. If it does, then the principle lying behind the approach suggests that the movement of resources should take place. The process is then repeated until no further shift of resources is worthwhile (in the sense of leading to a gain in total net benefit). Thus the economic approach is a combination of programme budgeting and marginal analysis with the key concepts being opportunity cost and the margin.

(I have sometimes suggested when teaching that if any of the participants falls asleep during my lecture and awakens conscious that I have asked a question but that it has gone unheard, then the best response is to mutter something about opportunity cost and the margin. This has something like a 50 per cent or higher chance of being at least partly right. In this particular case, opportunity cost and the margin say it all if the question concerns what are the key economic concepts in priority setting. It is worth emphasising this point as we will see later that very often methods used to set priorities omit one or both of these concepts.)

Programme budgeting is a simple mechanism for providing an information framework to assist the process of allowing resource use and outputs generated to be set alongside health service objectives and for helping to identify and begin the examination of relevant margins through marginal analysis. Programme budgeting is not evaluative in itself, but rather creates a framework in which evaluation is facilitated and encouraged.

In any health authority it will be possible to identify a series of broad programmes, for example, by disease group – cancer, respiratory disease, etc.; by client group – the elderly, mentally ill, etc.; or perhaps by geographical location. There is a range of possibilities. However the distinguishing feature of programmes is that they are 'output' orientated rather than 'input' orientated, as is the case with standard budgetary procedures. This is because, while the total spending on nurses (an input), for example, is an important piece of information in managing health services, the role of programme budgeting is to allow planning of health care and priority setting across different aspects of health care in ways that relate to the goals or objectives of health care. It is this 'objectives' orientation that requires programme budgeting to be output orientated.

More simply, it might be said that the designation of programmes ought to be such that all programmes can have health care objectives associated with them, which is clearly the case for maternity care or cancer therapy. It is this output and objectives orientation that distinguishes programme budgeting from other forms of budgeting.

(There is a form of budgeting called 'output' budgeting where the orientation is even more related to outputs than is programme budgeting. In an ideal world I would argue for this output budgeting in health care where the outputs might be defined in terms of various categories of health. But the information does not readily exist to get cost data in these terms nor does it exist with respect to the outputs. But it may be helpful to the reader to recognise that that would be the ideal route to go down if it were open to us.)

It is also potentially important that these programmes can be disaggregated into sub-programmes such as in the context of maternity care, ante-natal care, the labour/birth period, and post-natal care. For each programme and eventually each sub-programme, the task is to set out what is being spent on each and also what is being achieved with each. For the latter, while the most accurate and appropriate indicator of output should be used as possible, in reality it will often be some readily available (and hence very often rather imprecise) measure that will be used, such as occupied bed days or discharges or consultations. It may also be useful to do this for more than the most recent year for which data are available, and go back to establish what trend there has been over the last few years. Here much will depend on data availability and the precise purpose of the planning and priority setting exercise.

While there are various ways that these tasks might be accomplished, it would seem sensible to establish a programme group or programme management group for each of the programmes. These might comprise professional staff working with the patients in the programme group – doctors, nurses, etc., managers for the programme, information and finance staff, and perhaps lay representatives. How such groups are set up will again depend on the local circumstances, but some grouping into 'programme management groups' will certainly be needed to get the process working in practice.

There is a sense in which 'programme budgeting' is a misnomer. Budgeting normally relates to some future expenditure for which there is attached some sort of financial plan. But 'programme budgeting' normally relates to expenditure which has already occurred, and to that extent it might be more appropriate to call it something like 'programme expenditure review' – which is what an exercise using programme budgeting in Scotland was called in the late 1970s. Whatever the merits of one name over another, this process is called and has been called programme budgeting in the past and it would probably be confusing to change it now. So here at least I will stick with the programme budgeting nomenclature.

Having set up programmes and sub-programmes and estimated the levels of expenditures on these and the outputs from these for at least one year and perhaps more, the scene is set – we have the 'information framework' – to begin to consider marginal shifts in resources. In practice, it might be that particular programmes can be analysed on the margin without actually setting out the programme budgets as suggested above. However, it is my experience that the health service managers involved do not have a clear idea about what is contained within particular programmes nor any real idea of the size of different parts of the total expenditures within programmes. As a result they welcome the push that programme budgeting provides to specify the contents of programmes and to 'get a handle on' the sizes of the expenditures involved in fairly broad terms in both programmes and sub-programmes.

It is also the case that the designation of programmes, and just as much sub-programmes, is a particularly important aspect of the process. This is because every division of the cake, be it between programmes or within programmes, constitutes a possible 'boundary' across which resources may be moved. It is likely to be in the same terms that the margins will be defined when marginal analysis is undertaken. I had an interesting experience working with programme management groups in Liverpool, where the issue of designating sub-programmes was a real problem but once solved provided a very good basis for identifying useful margins for considering shifts in resource use. (For a more detailed look at programme budgeting, see Mooney *et al.*, 1986; and Mooney *et al.*, 1992.)

Marginal analysis is used when, having established the programme and sub-programme budgets, there is a requirement to look at how resources might be better deployed. It thus addresses the following three issues:

1. If there are no more resources available, can, say £1 million be moved from programme X to programme Y and the overall total benefit be increased?
2. If more resources are made available, on which programme or

sub-programme are these additional resources best spent in the sense of creating most extra benefit?

3. If expenditures are to be cut, where should the cut occur so that the impact in terms of loss of benefit is minimised?

The theory underlying this approach is simple. On the margin of each programme or sub-programme, for some fixed size of budget allocated across the whole set of programmes, the optimal allocation of the budget occurs where the ratio of marginal benefit to marginal cost is the same across all programmes or sub-programmes.

The details of how this is arrived at are provided in Mooney *et al.* (1986) but what it amounts to in practice can be explained simply (as indicated on p. 27). If it is possible to move £Z from A to B and as a result increase the overall total benefit (i.e. the gain in B is greater than the loss of benefit in A), then this represents an improvement in efficiency and as such should be done. Such moves should continue until it is the case that no further movement of funds will result in still greater benefits being provided. When this stage is reached with respect to all programmes, i.e. it is not possible to provide still greater benefits unless more resources *in toto* are provided, that is the optimal situation with respect to efficiency.

In practice the process will probably involve programme management groups for each programme working within each programme first and looking at margins across the sub-programmes. It is here that the nature of the divisions into sub-programmes is particularly important as it is these divisions which dictate to a large extent the nature of the margins analysed. Ought £100,000 to be taken from the ante-natal programme and spent in the post-natal programme? Should more resources go to screening older women in pregnancy even if younger women as a result get fewer resources spent on them during their pregnancies?

The margins across programmes will then be considered in a similar fashion once the individual programmes have been assessed and analysed. At this level – the cross-programme level – the decisions and judgements will be made presumably by the highest authority in the management of the services as a whole. Such decisions at this level will be much more 'political' and are likely to be quite heavily influenced in practice, depending on the precise nature of the health care system, by politicians themselves.

In practice, there may be a need for an intermediate step between the setting of the programme budgets and the marginal analysis. To perform the marginal analysis 'properly' requires that those who are exercising the judgements about what the benefit gains and losses are for the shift of the £Z, need to know what the benefits and the costs are of a potentially very wide range of options for change. Now in practice, they may know neither! With respect to benefits, ideally they might move in the direction of trying to establish a QALY league table or some health gain or benefit gain league table (see Chapter 4). Certainly, any step in this direction will be useful, but it is as well to recognise that in the current state of the art, any assessment of benefit will be highly subjective. Of course, there is no way of removing totally the subjectivity involved in such choices – to trade off health gains for the elderly versus health gains for children has to be subjective. But there may not be very good information available even on the technical issue of the likely impact on health of various ways of using the extra monies. This has to be accepted and overcome to the extent that available analytical resources or the existing literature on effectiveness will allow.

The same problems exist, of course, when there is a need to think about reductions in various programmes or sub-programmes. Again, there may at best be poor information about the benefit losses likely to occur in these circumstances.

It is also unlikely that there will be a lot of information readily available about the marginal costs of the various changes that might be considered as possibles for shifting resources. There are likely to be data about average costs, and while there will be a great temptation to use these, the chances are very strong that the use of these average cost figures will lead to the costings being wrong. It is not that we can automatically assume that average costs will be different from marginal costs, but to assume that they will be different rather than assuming that they will be the same is a much better starting point!

Many costing studies would thus be needed and this in itself could be a very big exercise. Note too that if those who are to perform the marginal analysis, the programme management groups, are to do it well, they will need cost data on all possible marginal changes that they might conceivably consider and someone has to guess in advance what these might be. In the event, it is quite likely that the programme management groups will not use more than a small proportion of the cost figures that have been worked out.

To avoid this long and time-consuming process, which could tie up the relatively few staff available for conducting analyses for the priority-setting exercises as a whole, this stage of the procedure is split into three. First, the programme management groups are asked to draw up 'wish lists' but without having good data available either on benefits or on costs. These will contain their best guesses about what the activities are that they would most like to see if more resources were made available to their programme or their sub-programmes (the 'incremental wish list') and similarly those activities they would be least reluctant to stop if they had a cut in their allocation of resources (the 'decremental wish list'). Second, these wish lists would be costed and assessed in more detail with respect to the impact each listed option would have on benefits. Third, the programme management group would perform the marginal analysis proper where they would assess the impact of shifts of resources of certain amounts, such as £100,000, as they would then have the necessary cost data to do this and as good information as could be made available on the benefit effects.

Clearly, with this approach, there is a possibility with the split into this three-way process that some important options could be missed. This is most likely to be the case on the initial wish list for low-benefit options which ought to have been included because they are also low-cost. For high-benefit, high-cost options this is less of a risk since there is likely to be, if anything, a bias on the programme management group towards letting perceived benefits rather than perceived costs determine the wish lists.

Overall, however, the risks seem worth taking, otherwise the whole exercise could get very heavily involved in costing studies, which might in turn make the process seem unworkable. Warning programme management groups of the likely bias in their assessments when drawing up wish lists can reduce the risk of serious omissions from their listings.

This 'economics approach' does require data on costs and benefits and it requires that these data relate to changes on the margins of programmes and sub-programmes. To that extent it might be claimed that the approach is data intensive (see p. 25 above). However, I would respond with two arguments. First, *any* system of priority setting will be data intensive. And second, I simply cannot see how efficiency of resource use can be pursued in practice without information about marginal costs and marginal benefits. Any approach to priority setting that does not involve some assessment of costs and benefits on the margins should, I believe, be treated with the utmost suspicion!

In the next section I shall begin to look at other approaches to priority setting and see these in the light of what I have written about the economic approach. However, before doing so I would want to highlight the fact that what has been said in this section deals only with efficiency – strictly, allocative efficiency. I have not covered equity. I discuss equity in detail in Chapter 5, but here it is worth saying that the best way to handle equity in priority setting is perhaps for it to be 'added on' at the end of the efficiency exercise. If the two – efficiency and equity – are considered together, then there is a risk that waters get muddied and there is a loss of clarity with respect to why particular options seem good or bad. Thus the best way to proceed might be as follows.

First, the authority responsible for the overall running of the services might make a clear statement about what their operational goal for equity is with respect to health, access or use. Thereafter, they might try (but it is difficult) to give guidance as to the relative weight to be attached to equity and in what dimensions – gender, social class and geographical location are the three fairly obvious ones. These equity guidelines would then be presented to the programme management groups to assist them in their deliberations, the idea being that they concentrate initially on efficiency concerns but then indicate what the equity impact would be of their various possible strategies.

When the choices overall come back to the main health service authority from the programme management groups, the final trade-offs between equity and efficiency would be made. Given the inevitably political nature of these choices, it would seem appropriate that these choices with respect to equity are made at this high level.

Priority setting: some existing approaches

A number of different approaches are found to priority setting in health care. These vary from country to country. However, most seem to come under the rather broad heading of 'needs assessment', or variants on this. Here I want to look at needs assessment; target setting as an increasingly popular variant of needs assessment; briefly at the use of 'severity', as adopted in Norway, as the key criterion of priority setting; QALY league tables (these are dealt with at greater length in Chapter 4) and cost of illness studies. These approaches are reviewed here not with the intent of being comprehensive, but to outline what the main approaches seem to be.

Needs assessment

The most common approach to priority setting would appear to be what is normally referred to as 'needs assessment'. This comes in various guises but in essence involves an attempt to assess the 'total needs' for health care for a population as a whole, or for a particular disease group, or a particular client or age group. This leads into priority-setting exercises which are initially concerned with assessing the needs for child health services, or for cancer patients, or for elderly people, and perhaps in aggregation of the people as a whole living in a particular location. It is particularly common in the United Kingdom at the time of writing, although happily there does seem to be a movement away from the total needs assessment approach to priority setting for purchasing in the NHS.

One needs to be cautious in writing about some of these issues and not set up strawmen. That would be pointless, but there is an argument for trying to distinguish between the principles involved in different approaches. They do not all get us to the same place and it ought not to be the case that we simply set out a stall with four or six or whatever number of approaches to priority setting and ask potential purchasers to enter this market and decide on the basis of their informed choice what methods to use. The potential buyers here, I would submit, are not informed. They need help and guidance. Some things are better than others; some need more effort and hence cost more than others. Some shortcomings are important; others are not. There is a sense in which this account might most usefully be interpreted as some sort of *'Which?'* consumer guide to priority-setting techniques.

The principle lying behind this approach seems to be that the total needs for health care can be established and that somehow this will provide a basis for setting priorities. What is not clear, however (at least to this observer), is what one does with the information on needs assessment. If one can establish the total needs for child health care, how do we move forward from that to establish priorities? If the needs for children aged 0 to 1 are greater than for those aged 1 to 2, what does this mean for the allocation of resources between these two groups? If the needs are twice as great, does this mean that resources should be allocated *pro rata* with the size of the relative needs? Are all needs in this sense equally weighted? In fact, before we can address these sorts of question we need to establish what is meant by need in this context.

There are two possibilities which in practice do not seem always to be distinguished as well as they might be. Yet they are different in principle and can be very different in the results that they provide. The first is that need can be directly related to illness or sickness. The more sickness there is in a population, the greater is the need (presumably for health care). Such a view of need would suggest that needs assessment would involve establishing a sickness profile, covering *inter alia* the incidence and prevalence of diseases in the relevant population. It would also be independent, at any moment, of the technological ability to deal with sickness (except in so far as it already had done so in some past time period).

Second, there is the view that need is about capacity to benefit. The greater the capacity to benefit from health care in a community the greater is the need in that community. Here there is now greater recognition of the fact that not all diseases or conditions can be 'cured' or their sufferers returned to 'full health'. There is also an implicit recognition that some diseases or conditions may be more amenable to treatment than others. This approach also embraces the notion that need is a function of existing technology. If the technology does not exist to deal with a disease or condition, no need exists under this approach (although there would be under the first definition of need).

There could be agreement under certain circumstances between the two approaches with respect to the relative amount of need for health care for various diseases. However, these conditions are fairly stringent and assume that all diseases are equally amenable to treatment. One observation that seems very relevant here to the appropriateness of this needs-based approach is that presumably at some stage of the proceedings there is a need to aggregate needs. If the desire is to establish the total need for, say, cancer services, then the needs for care for different cancers presumably have to be established and in some way aggregated. This presumably is also true *within* categories of cancers. For example, there may be a need to establish the need for care for breast cancer for women in different stages of the disease or in different age or risk groups.

But how is this aggregation to be done? Under the first essentially sickness approach it means adding together the amounts of sickness. But how are these different amounts to be added together? One possibility is to establish some sort of indicator, which would reflect the amount of health gain in the community if diseases were *eradicated*. This might be in terms of something rather crude like years of life lost prematurely from a disease (as is done in e.g. *The Health of the Nation*, DoH, 1992). Or it might involve an estimate of the 'burden of disease' in terms of, say, 'total QALYs lost from breast cancer' or 'total QALYs lost from breast cancer among women aged 40 to 50'. It might adopt some sort of 'cost of illness' calculation where the burden of the disease in terms of sickness might be added to the cost of treatment and the costs of lost output in the economy as a result of the disease's existence. But while the literature is not always clear on this point, some measure of need is required and it is presumed here that that measure has to be something to be related in some way to the burden of disease.

Under the second approach there is greater clarity with respect to what is involved. Since need here is classed in terms of capacity to benefit (Culyer, 1991) need can be measured in terms of the health gains that will be achieved if the disease condition is treated as fully as possible, i.e. until the marginal productivity of treatment has fallen to zero. We do not have the burden of disease *per se* but the burden of disease that is potentially removable, given current technology. If there were technologies which were 100 per cent effective for all conditions, then the two measures would be identical.

One thing to note in passing about these two approaches is that to operate effectively they both need some assessment of the benefits of a whole variety of treatments. They thus require that such benefits be measurable. I mention this here to emphasise the point that it is not just the economics approach that needs a measure of benefit. However at the same time, at least up to this point, they do not require any measure of cost. Consequently, in terms of ease of application the two needs assessment approaches are easier to apply.

The total needs assessment approach, where the total burden of disease is estimated, seems so inappropriate that it will not be discussed further here. It entails *inter alia* setting priorities on the basis of the size of a problem whether there is any possibility of dealing with it or not. (It is the true burden of illness approach as outlined later in this chapter.)

The second approach to needs assessment is preferable. Here it is accepted that not all illnesses can be cured, indeed that illnesses are curable or treatable to varying extents. It is here that the concept of capacity to benefit comes into consideration. The technological constraints are accepted. This clearly is a move forward.

However, such an approach still leaves us with the question: having estimated for various diseases the total needs in terms of capacity to benefit, and assuming we have a measure that allows us to state what these needs are in some commensurable measure across various very different diseases, what do we do with the information? (I will come back to the issues of measurement again below.)

There seem to be various possibilities but they can only be possibilities since it is here that the process seems finally to break down. I can find nothing in the literature which indicates what the needs assessors would do with the information – at least in a way that I would consider is directly relevant to priority setting.

One possibility is to argue that resources should be allocated *pro rata* with needs. The logic here would be that since this form of needs reflects capacity to benefit, then allocating resources in this way would maximise the amount of need met. But resource use has to reflect the costs of treatment. What about the costs of meeting the needs? It would only be if the cost per unit of need met (perhaps health gain) were constant across all diseases and conditions, and that for all these diseases and conditions average and marginal cost were equal, that this use of the estimates of needs assessed would be valid. That is most unlikely to hold good. Put another way, it would mean that all diseases could be treated in an equally operationally efficient way, i.e. that all diseases were equally cost effective in their treatment. It would require further that technological developments in medicine and in the delivery of health care were such that they did not affect the cost-effectiveness of such treatments at all. It would additionally mean that there were no economies (or diseconomies) of scale for any disease or condition.

A second possibility would be to argue more basically that the needs assessments should be used simply as an ordinal ranking, i.e. that the disease with the greatest needs should get more resources than that with the next greatest need, and so on. In some ways this is more appealing. However, if the cost effectiveness of interventions varies, then again there is no reason to think that the greatest need should be given priority. Further, if we adopted this ordinal ranking, how would it be used? At what point would we say: that is enough spending on the top need, now let us move to the next? In other words, the lack of cardinality leaves us unable to use the margin in resource allocation decision making.

A third possibility is to use the needs assessment information in some form of weighting process, which might reflect priorities. Thus if it were felt that those diseases or conditions that created the most need in society should be given priority over and above any considerations of some simple cost-effectiveness criterion of allocating resources in such a way as to maximise health gains, then the ranking of needs assessment could be used to arrive at weights. Thus if, say, cardiovascular disease were the disease for which there was the greatest need, then the health gains from any interventions which had an impact on reducing the needs there might be weighted more highly than those for interventions on other diseases which came further down the needs league table.

Such a system still leaves open the question of how the ordinal ranking would be converted into cardinal weights. More fundamentally, there does seem some sort of 'big problem' imperative in much of health policy. Yet there is little logic in the notion that simply because the disease that I suffer from happens to be a common one, that that by itself and *ceteris paribus* should mean that I get higher priority for treatment than someone suffering from a rather less common disease. Yet this would be but one rather illogical result of weighting by size of need.

This 'size of the problem' imperative is also present in cost of illness-based priority setting (as discussed later in this chapter). It is perhaps understandable that policy makers might be attracted by the approach at a superficial level, but I cannot see how the approach survives any detailed scrutiny.

Beyond concerns about how the data on needs assessment might be used, there is the question of how the information might be presented. In other words, if attempts are made to assess the relative needs of, say, cancer and cardiothoracic disease, or even, and more closely together, the needs of breast cancer sufferers versus those of lung cancer sufferers or even breast cancer sufferers at different stages of the disease, there has to be a mechanism or measuring rod for adding together the needs within categories and a means of comparing these totals across these different categories of disease. Presumably the needs assessors would use some sort of measure of health gain, or just benefit. However, within the needs assessment literature there is a strange and rather empty silence on this issue. Perhaps that is understandable. The point is made here not strictly by way of criticism but more simply to emphasise that the measurement problems discussed here are rather similar to the measurement problems in the economics approach to priority setting. It would have to be admitted, however, that they are still greater under the economic approach, in essence because the economic approach requires the benefit measure to be on the margin and does not assume the constancy of average and marginal that needs assessment does. It also requires data on costs which the needs assessment method appears not to require.

On this issue of cost and priority setting it may be that it is less than clear to some readers why costs are needed in setting priorities. This is because of the concept of opportunity cost (as mentioned on p. 27). Priority setting is about working out where best to allocate scarce resources, and forming that judgement needs an assessment not only of the benefit of one intervention over another but also an assessment of the costs – the benefits forgone – elsewhere.

If we do not allow for costs in priority setting, then this would mean that if some new technology allowed heart transplants to be carried out at one tenth of their current cost, then such a change would have no effect on priorities in health care. Again, if the costs of hip replacements rose sixfold, would this not have an effect – should this not have an effect – on the level of supply of hip replacements?

Needs assessment leaves this observer wondering what there is to gain from any assessment of needs as a totality. It is possible (as discussed in greater length in Chapter 5 on equity) that a case can be made for assessing total need in the context of equity. There is no case for total needs assessment exercises for promoting allocative efficiency. They are at best irrelevant to the issue to hand; at worst they may create the illusion that total needs are capable of being met. More subtly and perhaps more dangerously still such exercises may result in allocations of scarce resources *pro rata* with assessments of total needs for resources for different diseases. This may get closer to where we want to be, but still ignores questions of the relative effectiveness and cost of interventions on the margin. It is here on the margin and with its lack of concern for costs that needs assessment fails as a helpful device for rational priority setting.

Needs assessment is based on faulty logic – the faulty logic of the imperative of the 'size of the problem'. That faulty logic needs to be exposed – and exposed again. It is so pervasive in health care. The fact that it is pervasive, however, is no reason for believing that it is in any sense right.

Before leaving needs assessment it is perhaps worth considering another phenomenon of needs assessment which may help to explain its popularity, at least in part. Certainly in the United Kingdom at present – and, I think, in many other countries – there are various planning and purchasing exercises which start with needs assessment. One of the potentially great advantages for needs assessors is that while they are engaged in such exercises, they do not have to face up to the difficult and demanding choices involved in priority setting of services: which services to expand and, more difficult, which services to cut? Which patients to refuse? Which patients to deny life to? Caught up in the apparently laudable task of assessing needs, the key choice that is required is what data to collect. This is not to mock the needs assessors. They are human, and making difficult, potentially tragic, choices is something that most of us would want to shy away from. It is easy for the economist who does not have to make the choices to promote the merits of explicit rational choice. For the decision makers such choices can raise difficult moral issues. There is process disutility here.

Adopting a sympathetic stance to those who have to make these tragic choices, however, is not the same as accepting that they should not be faced. If they are so difficult, then societies should more readily accept that and invest in more training of those who have to make them. I recall many years ago asking a cancer specialist why it was that there seemed to be a moral imperative on oncologists to treat disease rather than patients. She replied: 'Lack of moral fibre'. A harsh judgement perhaps, but that doesn't make it any less accurate.

Explicit choices – even if they are tragic ones – need to be made in health care if priority setting is to help us arrive at efficient solutions in resource allocation. If needs assessment is part of the process of keeping our distance from difficult choices, then there is a need to provide better training and create appropriate incentives to get decision makers to face the choices explicitly. The dividends from such explicit choices are great and in my view more than enough to justify the extra investment in training and organisational changes which might be required to get decisions faced and to overcome the lack of moral fibre that may hinder better decision making in health care and which lends support to the needs assessors. (The issue of getting economics used more in health care is addressed in greater detail in Chapter 12.)

Target setting

There is in itself little wrong with the idea of setting targets in priority setting. Indeed, targets can provide incentives for action and the issue of incentives more generally is one that is somewhat neglected in priority setting. However, very much depends on how the targets are set, and it is here that reservations have to be expressed. The experience to date is not encouraging.

The most famous, or notorious, targets in health and health care are those set by the World Health Organisation (WHO) in their pursuit of the goal of Health For All in the Year 2000. These are in essence largely challenges rather than anything more substantial. They are a mixture of concerns for better health; greater equity especially across countries; a desire to involve all sectors of the economy in the provision and promotion of health and not just the formal health care sector; and a large dose of exhortation. Whether they succeed or not remains to be seen, although as a source of propaganda for health there can be little doubt that they have been effective. What their impact on health will have been by the year 2000 we will not know, as no form of monitoring of any valid type as far as I am aware has been set up to answer the question of whether the Health For All strategy will have been an efficient one, or even an effective one.

The targets in themselves are fairly harmless. However, the long-term impact may well have been deleterious on three fronts. First, for those countries well below the targets when they were set – Hungary as compared to Sweden, say – there may well have been a concern that there was a lack of understanding in WHO about the differences in all sorts of cultural and economic phenomena which these two countries faced. (See, for example, Angelus (1990) on the Hungarian position *vis-à-vis* the WHO targets.) This could well have had the effect of depressing morale among Hungarian policy makers – the exact opposite of what the target setters intended.

Second, others have followed in the steps of WHO and gone for target setting as a vehicle for health policy. However, at a national level the sorts of target setting that may have been appropriate for WHO are less likely to be so for a national government which has at least some executive power to influence what actually happens on the ground.

Third, and in a sense related to the last point, the WHO targets are in essence part of their propaganda and sloganising for health. They do not have to take responsibility for their implementation. Among national governments such as that in the United Kingdom in their policy strategy *The Health of the Nation* (DoH, 1992) adopting the sloganising approach may well prove counter-productive. There is a responsibility at that level to go beyond slogans and consider operational planning of health care. As a result of the WHO target-setting bandwagon, increasingly it seems governments are stepping back from health care policy-making. They set targets and then leave those at the lower echelons of policy making to determine how the targets are to be reached.

This is heady and indeed very dangerous stuff, because it means that objectives are set without due consideration of means. Goals may be too expensive to achieve. Resource considerations are not included in the process of target setting. It is words without due consideration of the actions necessary to make the words fulfilling.

Targets are, or ought to be, about allocative efficiency and equity. (And with respect to the latter, some of WHO's targets *are* related to equity.) But at the level of allocative efficiency, as has been stated throughout this chapter, objectives, and thereby allocative efficiency, have to be pursued, taking due account of costs and benefits on the margin. If this is not done, it is difficult to see – I would say impossible – how allocative efficiency can be advanced with any certainty. If this process is not adopted in target setting, then there is a very real danger that the targets not only fail to further efficiency but may actually promote inefficiency. In other words, it is not just that they are not 'perfect', they will not be even an approximation to perfection. They are not an approximation in principle, so it is difficult to see how – but for chance – they can result in an approximation in practice in what they can actually achieve.

As an example of the target-setting approach in practice, let us examine briefly *The Health of the Nation*, which was the UK government's attempt to introduce the concept of target setting explicitly into health care planning and priority setting. In fact, this was an example not just of target setting but a form of needs assessment as well.

The process involved in determining at a national level what services were to get high priority ('key area' status in the language of the document) used three criteria for determining that an area was 'key'.

First, there had to be a big problem in terms of health, or more accurately, illness. This seems to be a form of needs assessment but of the first type outlined above, i.e. a big health problem, whether there is capacity to benefit or not.

Second, if that test were passed, there had to be effective interventions (although, beyond the very obvious, just what this means is not very clear from the document). However, on the face of it this would seem to result in a shift to the second form of needs assessment outlined above. (Note though that a small problem with the availability of very high effective interventions which might well pass the test of considerable ability to benefit would be screened out in the first round here, on the basis that it was not a big problem.) And third, there had to be the possibility of setting quantified targets in the area. Pass all three and an area was deemed to be high priority.

The sorts of criticism that can be made to this approach will be obvious to the reader, given what has been said earlier in this chapter: there is no consideration of costs; there is no consideration of the margin; there is no consideration of the benefits, except in a rather loose way; and there is no consideration of the weighing up of costs and benefits on the margin. It is sloganising for health in the sense of saying: let's get rid of the big health problems; rather than: let's maximise the health of the nation.

There is no reason at all to believe that the approach will promote allocative efficiency. Consequently, there is no reason to believe that within the resource constraints imposed it will achieve the greatest health possible for the nation.

It is perhaps worth re-emphasising that I do not mean to criticise target setting *per se*. If targets were set on the basis of weighing up costs and benefits on the margins – as they could be – then I can see considerable merit in them. Certainly, one would want to allow for variations at the local level, and advice and guidance would be needed at the local level about how to use the targets sensibly and flexibly. But that is the key merit to target setting, i.e. this visibility in where we want to go, with the visibility allowing goals to be shared, striven for, and so on. But the targets in the *Health of the Nation*, and the targets that are most frequently used in health care, do not embrace the marginal cost versus marginal benefit principle, so they fail to promote allocative efficiency. It is possible to get the advantages of target setting tied to the advantages of the pursuit of allocative efficiency. Indeed that is the challenge.

The Health of the Nation fails the most important challenge of all. It is sloganising for health on the basis of the big problem imperative. It is an opportunity missed to lead the local planners down the road of effective purchasing. (And while these comments are particularly germane to the United Kingdom they are also relevant elsewhere, not least since other countries may be adopting a similar approach, as is happening, for example, in the Department of Health in New South Wales, Australia.)

Severity as a criterion for priority setting

An interesting example of another approach to priority setting is provided by the Lønning Committee Report in Norway (NOU, 1987). This advocated that priorities should be set according to 'degree of severity of conditions'. There are five such categories, top of the list being people who will die in the short run, then down the list through various more mild conditions.

The idea is an interesting one and has some relationship to priority setting according to triage, which has been used on battlefields to decide on priorities for treating the wounded. Here the wounded are placed in one of three categories: those who are seriously injured and are going to die whether they receive treatment or not; those who are less seriously injured and will recover even if not treated; and those who will recover, or recover faster, if treated. It is the last category that is given priority.

However, triage does seem to have one important advantage over Lønning. Lønning looks only at severity, whereas triage takes account of the impact of intervention. In other words, the severity index in triage is adjusted to look at what the benefits are likely to be, rather than simply assuming, as in Lønning, that interventions will be of equal effectiveness. The fact that someone is close to death is seemingly a sufficient reason under Lønning for that person being placed in the top category for treatment. Whether he or she might die anyway is ignored.

Lønning also ignores the question of cost. If it is the case that one intervention is more costly than another, then *ceteris paribus* this should count against the more expensive intervention. This follows directly from the logic of scarcity of resources, but is not addressed in Lønning (nor seemingly in triage, although it is likely that resource intensity will be taken into account at least in some rough and ready way in triage). Lønning also fails to allow for any concept of the margin, and the appearance is of a lexicographic ordering such that all

the individuals who are in category 1 are treated ahead of any in category 2, and so on. There is no concept of diminishing marginal benefit here nor of possibly increasing marginal costs.

Such criticisms mean that Lønning is not an acceptable way of assessing priorities. Indeed, it is an example of how, from an economic perspective, one can ask the following questions of an approach and, if the approach 'fails the test', one can then argue that it will not provide an appropriate basis for efficient resource allocation through priority setting of that form. The questions are:

1. Does the approach incorporate some assessment of the cost of interventions?
2. Does the approach incorporate some assessment of the benefits of interventions?
3. Is the approach operating on the margin?

If the answer to even one of these questions is no, then the approach is suspect if efficiency is the goal of priority setting.

QALY league tables

It is appropriate in a chapter on priority setting to consider QALY league tables and their strengths and weaknesses. These issues, however, are dealt with at length elsewhere (see Chapter 4) and in Gerard and Mooney (1993). Here I want briefly to reiterate the key points made there with respect to these league tables. These are that they do embrace many of the principles that ideally I would like to see in priority setting. They are based on the idea of weighing up costs and benefits on the margin and to that extent are to be encouraged and recommended for priority setting. However, certain reservations need to be expressed about the way in which they are built and the limitations in their use.

First, they tend to be based on studies and study results drawn from an illegitimately wide geographical location. Since they are about what to do with extra resources on the margin, they ought to be specific to that issue in whatever location priority setting is to be helped by these study results.

Second, since they incorporate the concept of costs per QALY as the basis of priority setting, they can only handle priority setting in these terms. This means that they do not allow goals other than health maximisation to come into the picture and they do not allow consideration of the use of other resources than those earmarked for health, which means that they are restricted on the cost side to health service resources. They cannot legitimately bring in resource use outside the health service, say by patients and their families or by other social services.

Cost of illness studies

There is a substantial literature on cost of illness studies where at least a part – and normally a major part – of the defence for doing these studies is that they can be used as a basis for setting priorities. Cost of illness normally covers the costs of treating the illness together with the costs (for example, from absence from work) arising as a result of the illness. The logic appears to be that if the costs of a particular illness are high as compared with another illness, then the higher-cost illness should get higher priority.

I do not agree with the logic behind this view. In fact, I think the depth of thinking underlying cost of illness studies, or 'the burden of disease' as it is sometimes called, as a basis for setting priorities is minimal. Yet their popularity seems to remain undiminished despite various critiques that have been made of the approach (see, for example, Shiell *et al.*, 1987; Davey and Leeder, 1993).

Briefly, however, we can look at cost of illness studies as a basis for setting priorities, and question them as we did above in the context of the Lønning Committee's approach to priority setting.

The three questions and answers in setting priorities through cost of illness studies are as follows:

1. Does the approach incorporate some assessment of the cost of interventions?

The answer is a qualified yes. Costs clearly are included in cost of illness studies but they are wider than just costs of interventions and they do not first consider issues of which interventions are being appraised.

2. Does the approach incorporate some assessment of the benefits of interventions?

The answer is a definite no. Cost of illness studies do not look at the issue of interventions *per se* and as a result the question of what benefit arises from different interventions is not tackled.

3.   Is the approach operating on the margin?

The answer here is again a definite no. The cost of illness studies are about the total costs of illness and do not consider marginal costs. Since they do not consider benefits at all, they certainly do not address the issue of marginal benefits.

So cost of illness studies receive only a very muted yes to one of the three questions and a resounding no to the two others. Bearing in mind that one 'no' is enough to raise a concern about the appropriateness of some proposed approach to priority setting, cost of illness studies as a basis for priority setting fail the test!

What, then, can explain their popularity? That is difficult to answer. There is a superficial attraction, somewhat similar to that in the needs assessment approach, in allocating resources to 'big problems', but that is so superficial that it is difficult to see that that is the real explanation. Partly too it may be that big numbers look impressive, and it may be for this reason that the pharmaceutical industry seems so keen to fund cost of illness studies. I suppose if they can show that a disease for which they have a product that will reduce or ameliorate the disease 'costs a large sum', then this may be a useful advertising weapon. I do not know. I cannot think that policy makers would succumb to such an argument, yet it seems that many cost of illness studies are funded by the industry, so perhaps there is something in that argument.

It could also be that such an approach is seen to have the advantage of disease in priority setting in health care in developing countries worrying in this context is that the World Bank, or at least some senior members of the World Bank staff, seem to have fallen for this argument and are recommending the use of cost of illness and burden of disease in priority setting in health care in developing countries (Jamison *et al.*, 1993). This follows in the wake of an article from another member of the World Bank staff, who argued that, despite the problems with burden of illness as a basis for priority setting, it had the merit of being 'conceptually simple' (Barnum, 1987).

It is certainly my view that the use of cost of illness and burden of disease studies as a basis for priority setting in health care will not lead to an efficient allocation of resources, nor that this is a way of getting to something approximating to efficiency. As Davey and Leeder (1993) remark in a neat, dismissive and accurate phrase: 'To know the cost of illness is to know nothing of real importance in deciding what we should do about the illness.' Yet the authors from the World Bank are none the less advocating an approach to priority setting based on such cost of illness thinking. The implications for the use of the very scarce resources that developing countries have available for health care are worrying should these countries follow this advice, since it is not possible to see how this approach can possibly lead to an efficient allocation of their health care resources.

Conclusion

My intention in this chapter was to indicate a way in which the task of priority setting can be assisted through the use of an economics approach, involving programme budgeting and marginal analysis. I have also indicated that there are other approaches, but that these seem deficient in certain ways. Additionally, I have set out three questions to be posed of any proposed approach to priority setting, all of which have to be answered in the affirmative before it becomes possible to argue that the approach will support the goal of efficiency in priority setting.

I hope I have presented some useful insights into priority setting. I hope too that these will be useful both in persuading the reader that the economics approach does have something very positive to offer the priority setters and perhaps convince the reader also that other methods fall short in various ways.

If I have succeeded, then I am delighted. I remain somewhat surprised and sometimes a little depressed at how difficult it seems to be to get those concerned with priority setting in health care to accept the economics approach and at the same time to acknowledge the deficiencies of, for example, needs assessment.

I will return to the more general issue of trying to get economics used more in health care in the final chapter.

References

Angelus, T. (1990) Hungarian health care: a challenge to medical values? In U. J. Jensen and G. H. Mooney (eds) *Changing Values in Medical and Health Care Decision Making*. Wiley, London.

Barnum, H. (1987) Evaluating healthy days of life gained from health projects. *Social Science and Medicine*, **24**, 10, 833–41.

Culyer, A. J. (1991) Health, health expenditures and equity. Discussion paper 83, Centre for Health Economics, University of York, York.

Davey, P. J. and Leeder, S. R. (1993) The cost of cost-of-illnes studies. *Medical Journal of Australia*, **158**, 583–4.

Department of Health (1992) *The Health of the Nation*. HMSO, London.

Gerard, K. and Mooney, G. H. (1993) QALY league tables: handle with care. *Health Economics*, **2**, 59–64.

Jamison, D. T., Mosley, W. H., Measham, A. R. and Bobadilla, J. L. (eds) (1993) *Disease Control Priorities in Developing Countries*. Oxford University Press, Oxford.

Mooney, G. H., Russell, E. M. and Weir, R. D. (1986) *Choices for Health Care*. Macmillan, London.

Mooney, G. H., Gerard, K., Donaldson, C. and Farrar, S. (1992) *Priority Setting in Purchasing: Some Practical Guidelines*. NAHAT, Birmingham.

NOU (1987) The Lønning Committee: Guidelines for priority setting in Norwegian health care. Ministry of Health and Social Affairs, Oslo.

Shiell, A., Gerard, K. and Donaldson, C. (1987) Cost of illness studies: an aid to decision making? *Health Policy*, **8**, 317–23.

4

QALY league tables: the road to better priority setting?

Introduction

In recent years there has been an increased effort in health policy internationally to get to grips with priority setting in a more rational, scientific, objective manner. As part of this push for better priority setting and more science the idea of QALY league tables has developed (see, for example, Williams, 1985; Australian Institute of Health, 1991). These have sparked much interest among policy makers. Some might even argue that the use of such tables represents *the* way to go in setting priorities.

In this chapter I shall examine QALY league tables in some detail, not with a view to arguing that they represent the ideal way for determining priorities, nor to suggest that they are an inappropriate basis for setting priorities. The emphasis rather is one of caution. Priority setting is hard, and fraught with various difficulties and pitfalls. QALY league tables certainly avoid some of these pitfalls, but equally certainly they need to be used, if at all, with considerable care.

Some overselling of QALY league tables has occurred in recent years. I want to suggest here that that overselling may be dangerous and not just in the short run in getting priorities set inappropriately. In the longer run there is a risk of a backlash not just against QALY league tables *per se* but also more generally against rationality in health care priority setting and perhaps (if a somewhat more selfish thought from this health economist!) against health economics in general. There is a risk in overselling anything and a need to ensure that expectations with respect to the 'product' are realistic. It is these thoughts that dominated the writing of this chapter, which is based in part on some work that I did with Karen Gerard (Gerard and Mooney, 1993).

I have encountered some criticism in voicing concerns about QALY league tables, especially among some of my fellow health economists, who seem worried that negative remarks about the usefulness of the QALY league table, such as those I make below, may be counter-productive. I do not think this worry arises because they think my criticisms are wrong. Rather, the concern seems to be that, given how badly priority setting is currently done in health care and given, in their view at least, that QALY league tables – warts and all – will lead to a better world, let us be careful not to give the impression that QALY league tables are beset with problems. Clearly, the question of whether we continue as of now with poor priority-setting ideas and techniques (and see Chapter 3 for more detail on this), adopt QALY league tables as they are or wait until we have something closer to perfection is a matter of judgement. The difficulty I see in forming such a judgement is that we have relatively little information or empirical evidence on which to base these judgements.

The middle ground I am advocating here is not necessarily the optimal strategy. What that middle ground involves in essence is saying yes to QALY league tables with all sorts of 'large print warnings' about the sometimes fragile bases for the construction of such tables and fears of overuse and misuse. At the same time the middle ground accepts that what currently happens is rather unsatisfactory, that there is considerable room for improvement, and that improvement in the technique of QALY league tables is highly desirable. But it also states that at a policy level the principles underlying QALY league tables need to be better understood and applied more widely than is currently the case.

Finally, the middle ground argues strongly that far more important at this stage in the development of priority setting techniques, and in particular QALY league tables, than improving the QALYs or improving the tables is improving the thinking in priority setting. If there is one thing I would like to change in the armoury of thinking of policy makers, it is how they set priorities. It is getting across strongly to them the concepts of opportunity cost and the margin. Most policy makers in my experience do not have these concepts. Those who are exposed to them have little difficulty in understanding them and readily recognise their relevance to health care planning and priority setting. Some of those who do understand apply them, while others 'backslide', very often in the face of entrenched disciplinary thinking which has persisted in health care for many years but which none the less has been shown to have failed. This backsliding is unfortunate even if understandable. It should stop, and the only way to stop it is to sell the economic approach better and to continue to expose the deficiencies of other approaches.

The arrogance of an economist? Yes – and with no apology! For far too long health care planning has been run by those who do not understand the key concepts involved in priority setting, and I can see no reason for trying to defend their position when I am convinced that it is leading to less – and less valued – health in societies than can be the case with no increase in resources at all. While epidemiology is clearly an important discipline in health care planning, the *philosophy* of much of epidemiology is unhelpful when priorities have to be set. While the science of medicine is necessary for understanding disease and reactions of disease to treatments, there is little in the *philosophy* of medicine which is helpful to priority setting as a process. Other disciplines from the social sciences are also potentially helpful as aids to implementing good priority setting. But the key to good priority setting arises from the same source as the discipline of economics – that when there are insufficient resources to do all that we would like to do, then we have to choose how best to use these resources. That is how economics arose as a discipline, and it is from that fact that economics continues to take its lifeblood. Similarly – indeed, identically but more specifically – priority setting in health care exists because resources for health care are scarce and choices have to be made.

In the next section I set out what QALY league tables are. It is important to understand these correctly, especially as there does appear to be quite a lot of misunderstanding about what they are and what they can be expected to do and in what way. Thereafter I want to say something about how QALY league tables are constructed. In the next section I will attempt a balanced critique of QALY league tables, arguing in essence that they are useful but advising caution in how they are used and interpreted. Finally, I suggest ways which will allow greater and more helpful use of QALY league tables in priority setting in health care.

What are QALY league tables?

A QALY league table is a device or procedure aimed at allowing priority setting of health care programmes when these programmes are competing for limited resources, and choices have to be made about which programmes to implement and which to leave unimplemented. The 'league table' ranks different procedures according to the 'cost per QALY' of implementing these procedures. The resource allocation decision rule underlying the use of these tables is that programmes should be implemented on the rank order basis of ascending cost per QALY.

Strictly, QALY league tables are 'marginal health service cost per QALY gained league tables (given various assumptions about existing resource allocation and about the objectives that health services are trying to meet in their priority setting)'. Given such a wordy description, it is hardly surprising that their name has been reduced to something nice and simple like 'QALY league tables'. But it is worth looking at the longer title to see just what QALY league tables are.

First, the fact that QALY league tables are about marginal costs per extra QALY is important. First, because the issue arises: marginal with respect to what? In other words, from where are we starting? The answer to this question – to some extent reassuringly, but as it turns out rather frustratingly – is that we are starting from where we are. QALY league tables are based on answers to the question: given the current allocation of resources in a particular area, what are the costs involved in purchasing additional QALYs through the implementation of more of the various procedures that are currently available or through implementing some new procedures altogether? If, say, there is an extra £100,000 to spend on health care, what is the maximum number of extra QALYs that that can buy? In which procedures is it best to invest more?

It can be anticipated that the cost of buying extra QALYs in a programme will be a function of a number of factors but almost certainly one of these will be how much of that programme is already being performed. As more and more is invested in a programme, it is likely that the cost per QALY on the margin will rise. This is because it is logical and rational (and efficient) to treat those patients first where the return in terms of QALYs per pound spent is highest and gradually work down to patients where the cost per QALY is getting higher and higher. Those patients treated first will be those easiest to treat, or for whom treatment is thought the most effective. Thus as a programme expands, so the cost per QALY is likely to rise. (This need not always be the case depending on the scale of the programme since within certain ranges of the programme there could be reduced marginal costs per QALY.)

It follows that the contents of a QALY league table are a function of what is currently going on within the geographical area for which the priority setting is being done. If, say, a particular health authority has already implemented a sizeable programme of heart transplants, then *ceteris paribus* the marginal cost per QALY of more heart transplants is likely to be higher than in an area which is lagging behind in its heart transplant programme. This is because the first authority will already have given transplants to those patients who are 'good buys' for such a procedure, and will now be looking at those patients at greater risk and perhaps greater cost and lower effectiveness.

A related factor worth noting here is that it follows from this form of difference across different authorities that the same kind of issue arises *within* an authority as the scale of one or more activity changes. In other words, as more and more hysterectomies are done, for example, so the cost per QALY within that authority is unlikely to remain constant and will most likely rise. Thus if a QALY league table at one point in time within an authority suggests that the lowest cost per QALY lies in the hysterectomy programme, after the authority has invested, say, £100,000 in more hysterectomies, it will be necessary to recalculate the marginal cost per QALY for the hysterectomy programme. If the cost per QALY has changed, then the position of hysterectomies in the QALY league table may also have changed, with the result that if another £100,000 becomes available, it may not be hysterectomies that are now the 'best buy' for additional QALYs.

Thus the issue of 'comparison with what' in QALY league tables is important and needs always to be examined when attempting to use such tables in priority setting (an issue we will come back to below). What is worth noting in principle here is that immediately the emphasis is on the margin, so identifying the baseline becomes important. If the baseline shifts, then there is a need to check what the repercussions of this are for the cost per QALY calculations and hence the position of the procedure in the league table.

Second, the reason why recognition that QALY league tables are about marginal costs per QALY is important is that priority setting here is not about the choice between programmes *per se*. It is about changes in the scale of programmes. Indeed, most QALY league tables are about increments in resources for programmes, i.e. they deal with the question of how best to spend *additional* resources. This will now be obvious to the reader from what has been said above, but there is a distinct feeling in some discussions about priority setting and about the use of QALY league tables that the issue is choosing between programmes. It is not. It is about changing the scale of programmes.

A smaller point relates to the direction of change. Priority setting can take place against the background of three possible scenarios with respect to the budget allocations: increased budget; decreased budget; or fixed budget (but with scope for redeployment within the budget). In most situations the QALY league tables that are published appear to relate to the first issue, i.e. what to do with a higher level of spending. The distinction between these three scenarios may be important for the construction and use of QALY league tables. Depending on the shape of the cost per QALY function, as the scale of a programme changes it may be that the cost per QALY for incremental marginal changes will be different, and sometimes quite different from the cost per QALY for decremental marginal changes. Similar problems may arise when we are considering the purchase of more of a programme through the reduction in spending on another programme. While this is a fairly obvious and, I think, clear-cut issue – the importance of which is difficult to gauge as there is little empirical evidence – it would seem important that those who use QALY league tables are aware of the issue. It may be still more important for those involved in constructing QALY league tables.

Beyond the issue of the margin, another important aspect of QALY league tables is that they are about QALYs. Now while that is a rather obvious statement there is the question of the extent to which QALYs are an accurate and acceptable measure of what is to be measured here. The question becomes: are QALYs an adequate measure of health; or more accurately, given the marginal nature of such matters, are QALYs gained an adequate measure of health gains? I will deal later with the issue of whether there is more than health to be considered when assessing the benefits of health care resource allocation, so I will not consider the question in detail here. However, I think that in the context of QALY league tables it is likely to be the case that for policy making, the QALY is as good a measure of health as is available at the present time, and for most purposes in priority setting an adequate measure. (There are, I believe, some real advantages in using HYEs but these are more difficult to work with in practice, and while I think superior not demonstratively so superior as to justify the extra problems involved in both calculating and using them; see p. 12)

What is worth stressing is that QALY league tables are seen as particularly useful in making comparisons across programmes, essentially because the QALY is not programme-specific. It is this broad nature of QALYs that allows the QALY league table to be used in priority setting across surgical, psychiatric, dermatological, etc., programmes. If this generality is cast in doubt – as it has been – then much of the value of the QALY league table would disappear; indeed, it would simply be unworkable. However, and again coming back to reality, my view would be that we have nothing better for the present. Consequently, this criticism of QALYs is such that, while there is undoubtedly something in it, it remains the case that QALYs appear better than anything else we have at the moment.

QALY league tables also assume that all that is relevant in the pursuit of priority setting in health care is that QALYs are maximised, which means in turn that assuming that QALYs do adequately measure health, that health is maximised. In so far as other considerations come into play in deciding how best to allocate resources to health and within health care, then QALY league tables will inevitably be deficient. Thus as discussed in greater length in Chapter 2, if there are other forms of benefit that are relevant in allocating resources – such as information, the protection of autonomy, or whatever – then the use of QALY league tables will lead to some distortions of the 'true' priorities.

Further, QALY league tables are about efficiency – essentially allocative efficiency, i.e. maximising the additional benefit from the additional resources available. They say nothing about equity, except in so far as equity is assumed away by arguing that a QALY is a QALY is a QALY, no matter who receives it and assuming that equity is to be seen in terms of health and not in terms of access or of use. As discussed in Chapter 5, there is good evidence to suggest that equity is most frequently seen by policy makers in terms of access, and as such QALY league tables that say nothing about access cannot cope with equity in this form. Thus priority setting according to QALY league tables is likely to leave the issue of equity, at least as most commonly identified by policy makers, on the side.

It thus follows that the objectives of health care that are assumed in QALY league tables are purely those of allocative efficiency where the only form of benefit is health. Issues of other benefits and questions of equity are not incorporated in QALY league tables.

The objectives of health care as assumed by QALY league tables are also somewhat problematical on the cost or resource side. On the benefit side the only benefit allowed is health. This means that, in terms of allocative efficiency, the only form that cost can take legitimately is in terms of opportunity costs where the benefit forgone is in terms of health. The QALY league table allows the question to be posed: is it better to spend here or here when only health benefits are being assumed?

This seems a reasonable assumption, if we once accept that health care is only about health, for those resources which are within the health care budget. But there are other resources which we would normally want to embrace in any economic appraisal of health care. These would include, for example, the resources of patients and their relatives; those of other social services such as housing and education services; and so on. But these provide potentially not just health benefits but also other forms of benefit: for the patient, the family and friends, the time input to care might have been used in a very wide range of other activities from watching TV to climbing mountains; the education services could have been producing more or different forms of education; and so on. The point is simply that these resources from outside the formal health care budget are not restricted in their use and hence in their opportunity costs to health-inducing activities. It is then difficult, indeed impossible, within the constraints imposed by a cost–utility framework to consider non-health service resource use within a QALY league table. It is simply not possible to say that patient time is best spent on this or that treatment, since that judgement can only be made across a much wider range of activities to which that patient time might have been an input.

That means that QALY league tables have to be restricted on the input or resource side in a similar way to that in which they are restricted on the output side, i.e. to health and, with respect to resources, to health service resources which have no alternative use than the production of health.

Now these caveats and qualifications about QALY league tables and their use are important. However, they do not mean that we should then abandon QALY league tables in priority setting. They are not perfect. They do have problems. But then as spelt out in Chapter 3, so do all the existing approaches to priority setting. At least with QALY league tables some of the key principles of priority setting are adhered to. What does emerge from this discussion is that we need to understand fully what QALY league tables can and cannot do, and that when they are constructed and used they should be treated with caution. Interpretation is crucial.

If QALYs are accepted as an adequate measure of health, then what QALY league tables do is to allow policy makers to address the question of how best to use additional health service resources in such a way as to maximise health gains. With care and adequate inputs in terms of the results of appropriate studies, QALY league tables will also allow policy makers to consider where best to cut resources across different programmes, and in turn how best to redeploy resources within a given budget, again where the objective is to maximise QALYs. And that, despite falling short of an ideal approach to priority setting, is no mean achievement for any technique.

Constructing QALY league tables

One key lesson to emerge from the discussion above is that the construction of good QALY league tables has to be handled with care.

Table 4.1 Comparative cost–utility results for selected programmes.

Programme	Reported cost/ QALY gained in US$	Year published	Adjusted cost/ QALY gained in 1988–9 A$
PKU screening	<0	1970	0
Postpartum anti-D injection	<0	1977	2,173
Antepartum anti-D injection	1,200	1983	2,173
Coronary artery bypass surgery for left main coronary artery disease	3,500	1981	7,564
Neonatal intensive care, 1,000 to 1,499 g	2,800	1978	8,159
T4 (thyroid screening)	3,600	1977	11,463
Treatment of severe hypertension (diastolic >105 mmHg) in males aged 40	4,850	1976	16,773
Treatment of mild hypertension (diastolic 95–104 mmHg) in males aged 40	9,880	1976	34,087
Oestrogen therapy for postmenopausal symptoms in women without a prior hysterectomy	18,160	1979	48,396
Neonatal intensive care, 500 to 999 g	19,600	1978	57,112
Coronary artery bypass surgery for single-vessel disease with moderately severe angina	30,000	1981	64,883
School tuberculin testing programme	13,000	1968	68,415
Continuous ambulatory peritoneal dialysis	35,100	1980	83,957
Hospital haemodialysis	40,200	1984	96,156

Source: Australian Institute of Health. *Cervical Cancer Screening in Australia: Options for change.* Prevention programme evaluation series no. 2. Canberra: Australian Government Publishing Service, 1991.

Unfortunately, the evidence to date on how they are constructed in practice suggests that care has not been evident when these tables have been constructed. The tables have to be built on the basis of studies of cost–utility analyses of different procedures. One such example, which is based on studies conducted in several countries, is presented above (see Table 4.1) (AIH, 1991). But how was the table developed and how useful is such a table to, say, the policy makers in New Zealand or in New South Wales or in Norway or in Norwich?

In the previous section it was stated that the way to construct QALY league tables was to establish for various options which QALYs could be bought through an extension of existing programmes. It was also emphasised there that the marginal costs per QALY were inevitably a function of what was already being done. But such marginal costs per QALY are a function of other factors as well. For example, they will be a function of the existing or remaining patterns of disease in the area in question. They will also be a function of the way in which medicine is practised in the area. And we know that the same conditions are treated in very different ways in different areas and certainly across different countries. They will also be a function of the way in which health services operate and the relative prices of the different factors of production. It is likely, for example, that there will be variation in the mix of staffing involved in wards of the same specialty across different countries, or regions within a country, or even in neighbouring hospitals. For example, some health services tend to be more nurse labour-intensive than others. Some reward their doctors more highly than do others *vis-à-vis* other grades and types of staff. All these factors mean that what some given amount of expenditure will buy by way of inputs and hence by way of health varies from country to country, and area to area within the same country. This means that in terms of transferring the results of cost–utility studies from one country to another, or one region to another, there is cause for exercising considerable care.

Indeed, it may be argued that such a transfer is not appropriate and that it is the results of *local* cost-utility analysis (CUA) studies that should be used in the construction of any QALY league table. In other words, ideally each country, or region, or area, should construct its own QALY league table to reflect the conditions which that country, or region, or area, faces locally. Certainly, there is a sense in which that would be ideal, especially if one accepts that the valuation of QALYs may well and legitimately vary from one area to another. There is no reason to believe, for example, that the relative weights attached to length of life and all sorts of different forms of quality of life will be constant across different areas of a country, never mind across different countries. (In the context of the Australian study of screening for breast cancer, which had to use some of the results from an earlier Swedish study, I was asked whether Swedish women's QALYs were likely to be different from Australian women's QALYs. I couldn't answer the question, but I think it is important to try to answer it and other, similar questions.)

Perhaps this issue is best understood if it is put round the other way. If we were to accept that QALY league tables – the same QALY league table – could be used in Humberside, Hobart, Hamilton and Harare, then this would mean that all these places had the same priorities for health care, irrespective of how they were currently delivering services and independently of what they were already doing in allocating resources and of what the diseases were and their prevalence in these locations, and how illness and disease were valued in these areas. That seems a most unlikely scenario! There has been too little thought given to this non-transferability of CUA results from one location to another.

There may be situations where such a transfer is both possible and legitimate. This is more likely, for example, in the case of certain forms of drug therapy where the resource inputs may be very similar from location to location, and where the marginal and average costs may be similar. But clearly this would apply only to those diseases that existed in the two locations. And of course, there is the issue of considering how the drug therapies rank *vis-à-vis* other forms of intervention.

The message here would seem to be not to trust the transfer of results from one location to another until the conditions under which the original study was done are understood and compared with the local situation. Only if these conditions are seen to be reasonably similar should the results from elsewhere be used locally.

One of the major problems facing would-be users of QALY league tables is that even if the transferability issue were not a problem, the number of CUA studies actually conducted is small. In the period from 1980 to mid-1991, for example, in the English language, Gerard (1992) could find only fifty-one studies published in journals and various reports. She herself is careful to point out that there could have been more, but given the way in which she obtained the fifty-one, it seems unlikely that many were missed.

Thus, even if the issue of transferability were not a problem, there are many procedures which have not been subject to cost-utility examinations. But the position is worse. Gerard indicates that for her sample of fifty-one there is considerable variation in the way in which the studies were done, which means that some could not be used legitimately at all in constructing QALY league tables and many are simply incompatible with one another in terms, for example, of the ways that QALYs were calculated and costs included.

That is a rather sorry picture. And certainly, as I return to below, if real progress is to be made in using QALY league tables, we need many more CUA studies. The fact that the popularity of the technique is growing should mean that within a reasonable number of years many more studies will have been conducted. But we need *many* more, especially if the issue of transferability should prove to be as great a problem as I believe it is.

Are QALY league tables worth the candle?

It is clear, I believe, that the concepts of opportunity cost and the margin on which QALY league tables are based are the ones that are appropriate for priority setting. As such, and since this is not true of all the approaches advocated for priority setting in health care, this is a very clear bonus for QALY league tables. However, it is evident from what has been said above that there are problems with QALY league tables.

Should they be constructed? Should they be used? And if so, how and in what circumstances?

The most famous example of the use of QALY league tables arose in Oregon. The aim there was to produce a QALY league table for services provided under the state of Oregon's Medicaid programme. The story of Oregon is well documented elsewhere (see, for example, Dixon and Walsh, 1991). It remains the case that to have tried this experiment in the United States was a major innovation. Much of the criticism of the Oregon experiment, however, is specific to Oregon rather than to QALY league tables as such. I would therefore not want to use the Oregon experiment to add further criticism to QALY league tables as a device for setting priorities.

The key message that I would like to convey with respect to the use of QALY league tables in health care policy making is that there are advantages in using QALY league tables, but that these will be lost if they are not used with care. To date the extent to which there have been 'warnings on the packaging' about the problems of misuse and overuse has been too little. As a result there is a danger of policy makers getting things wrong using QALY league tables and for the future perhaps becoming disenchanted with the whole idea of QALY league tables and indeed rational approaches more generally to priority setting.

What would seem desirable is to try to test the extent to which it is possible to use some rather rough and ready QALY league tables at a local level, which are based on local studies and local data. It seems most unlikely that the QALY league table that is relevant to planning health care in New South Wales, for example, will be at all relevant to planning services in Greater Glasgow Health Board. Primarily, I suspect that the biggest problems of transferability lie in differences in what is currently done (i.e. the services currently being provided) and differences in the underlying morbidity and mortality. There are, however, as indicated previously, all sorts of other reasons why the transfer of CUA results from one location to another may well be illegitimate. And it is for these reasons that I would advocate local QALY league tables.

Given Gerard's findings – that there were only fifty-one CUA studies conducted in the English language in the 1980s, and that some of these were poorly done and the remainder were not on a common basis which would then allow the results to be incorporated into a QALY league table – to advocate local QALY league tables may be seen as the counsel of the impossible or even the ridiculous. How can local health authorities in different countries be expected to set up studies to allow the results to be fed into local QALY league tables?

Certainly, it appears an awesome task. But the point to be made is that rough and ready efforts at a local level are likely to be better than the use of apparently precise figures from other locations which are based on and drawn from circumstances which are very different from those in the area to which they are being transferred. I cannot prove that, but it does seem very dangerous for policy makers simply to look at some general QALY league table and give top priority in their own area to whatever is the least cost per QALY option in that table. The logic of that is that that programme should have top priority in all settings around the country or indeed around the world!

Of course, even trying to set up rough and ready QALY league tables based on local CUA studies and their results is a considerable task. Yet since currently there is so little evidence that the thinking underlying QALY league tables – opportunity cost and the margin – is being adopted, the issue of the accuracy of QALY league table calculations is somewhat academic.

One of the things that Gerard (1992) attempted in her review of CUA studies was to ask whether the use of CUA added to the value of a study as compared with a simpler cost-effectiveness analysis (CEA) study. Now she had only limited success in answering that question given the lack of information in published studies to allow the question to be answered. However, it is of note that for the thirty-seven studies where a judgement on this was possible, for less than two-thirds was there value added through using CUA as compared with CEA.

More evidence at this level would be useful in trying to devise ways of getting to local QALY league tables which would be sufficiently accurate for the task for which they are to be used. That would seem to be the acid test. Are they good enough? And I am prepared to guess that such tables can be devised without too great expense to allow this to be done.

What of QALYs themselves? While I am clear that there is a case for continuing research on QALYs and HYEs (see my comments in Chapter 2), in the specific context of priority setting I am not convinced that the top priority is improving QALYs. I do think changing the thinking of the policy makers concerned with priority setting is the key here.

Clearly, there is a need for many more studies using CUA to be conducted. It ought increasingly to be the case that clinical trials automatically have an economic evaluation attached to them. There are moves afoot at this level to try to improve the position, but the current attitudes of major funders in this area – for example, in the United Kingdom, the Department of Health and the Medical Research Council (MRC) – are not helpful. I have had firsthand experience of clinicians simply refusing to co-operate in economic evaluations. And I see the MRC adopting a less than even-handed attitude to clinical research as compared with economic research. That needs to change but will not until there is a much greater recognition that clinical trials are too important to be left purely to the clinicians. That will be accepted in time, but it is a slow process.

There is also a need to get the incentives right to interest economists in this field. Certainly, the pharmaceutical industry is paying close attention to economic evaluation, but they have the money to buy health economists – both to employ them and to get them to act as consultants from their academic positions. And to have clinical trials and economic evaluations conducted by the industry or at least funded by the industry when the industry have such vested interests in the results does not seem the most sensible way to fund clinical research. (However, the Australians have taken the lead here and are now requiring that new drugs be subjected to economic evaluation before they can be considered for the Australian market.) But in other clinical research the incentives are wrong, with economists having to fight to get in on the act and the funders not providing adequate support. That has to change if they are serious about the way in which clinical trials and economic evaluations are linked in the future.

Conclusions

QALY league tables handled carefully are useful in priority setting. What is needed to get them used more and better is that a programme of research linked to policy is conducted along the following lines:

1. It is necessary to establish what the state of the art of priority setting is at the present time. What *are* policy makers doing in setting priorities? What goals do they have? What techniques are they using? Are they familiar with opportunity costs and the margin? Do they know about QALY league tables, and are they using them? If not why not? And so on.
2. What can be done to get the use of CUA extended and to become virtually routine in all clinical trials? How can the clinicians be made to accept the need for economic evaluations? How can the

research funders encourage more work of this type? How can we get more economic researchers to work in this area?

3. Are rough and ready local QALY league tables possible? What is involved in devising them? How can the possible success of such rough and ready tables be tested? Who should take the initiative in such a task? How expensive would such an exercise be?

4. Can results be transferred from one area to another? Can any sorts of guidelines be devised to establish in what circumstances such transfer is legitimate or at least sufficiently legitimate to allow results from one area to be transferred to another area?

5. Can more testing be done to establish the sensitivity of QALYs with respect to where it matters and in what circumstances that CUA is used rather than CEA? In other words, is it possible to investigate what the value added is of moving from CEA to CUA? Can rough and ready QALY measures be used (where, for example, anything other than death or good health is scored as a half)?

This is not intended as a complete agenda. However given what is said in Chapter 3, there is scope for improving marginal analysis and programme budgeting as currently applied. One way to do this and without too much cost is to incorporate some QALY league table calculations which use perhaps some rather crude cost and QALY measures.

It is clear from what has been discussed in this chapter that we have a long way to go before QALY league tables get to the point of being adequate at a local level for the purposes for which they are intended. However, sticking to the principles underlying them seems crucial. Getting the policy makers and the economists together to assess what needs to be done in a pragmatic way to get the tables into an adequate form to be used and to be useful also matters. That seems the way to go, at least for the next few years – and maybe few here will turn out to be many!

So this is not a counsel of despair but rather a plea – yet again – for keeping to good principles and using initiative and ingenuity in manipulating data to allow the principles to be applied. That sort of thinking – good principles and pragmatism with data – seems to be emerging as one of the key features of this book!

References

Australian Institute of Health (1991) *Cervical Cancer Screening in Australia: Options for change.* Australian Government Publishing Service, Canberra.

Dixon, J. and Walsh, H. G. (1991) Priority setting: lessons from Oregon. *Lancet*, **337**, 891–4.

Gerard, K. (1992) Cost utility in practice: a policy maker's guide to the state of the art. *Health Policy*, **21**, 249–79.

Gerard, K. and Mooney, G. (1993) QALY league tables: handle with care. *Health Economics*, **2**, 59–64.

Williams, A. (1985) Economics of coronary bypass grafting. *British Medical Journal*, **291**, 326–9.

5

Equity

Introduction

Equity is one of the key objectives of most health care systems – at least in terms of various policy documents and policy statements it appears to be so. However, the reality, in terms of the extent to which equity is pursued in practice, is not always what one might conclude from reading the policy documents.

Most countries have some sort of statement about their equity policy, which is normally couched in terms of equality of access. However, there is considerable doubt, in some quarters, about what 'access' means in the context of equity in health care and whether access is a goal in itself or whether it is purely instrumental, with equality of health being the 'true' goal. Again, there are those who interpret access in terms of use, so that equal access becomes equal use, usually in the form of equal use for equal need. The position is not helped by the fact that in US English it seems that 'to access' means 'to use'! As far as I am aware, however, the language in this chapter is British English!

In what follows I shall examine the possible ways of looking at equity and consider what the implications for health policy are of adopting one definition or another. I shall also make the case for suggesting that the issue of definition is important. As Grossman and Leeder (1991) have written: 'If we don't agree on a definition of inequity, how can we work together to reduce it?' In similar vein Birch and Abelson (1992) state: 'From a policy perspective it is . . . important to specify precisely what is meant by equity; equity of what and among whom, in order to derive appropriate policy conclusions for pursuing equity goals.'

What emerges in this chapter is that there can be no uniquely right or wrong position or definition with respect to equity in health care. At least, there can be no right or wrong definition which is independent of some view of what society is about or what health care is about with respect to certain distributional goals. Once the goals are clearly stated then there are positions which are not so much right or wrong as consistent or inconsistent. (I will have quite a lot to say about consistency as I think that this distinction between what is right and what is consistent is not made as often as it might be, and that as a result of this failure, the equity debate sometimes gets rather confused and confusing.) What any concern for equity has to start from is a view of what a just distribution of health, or health care, is.

I address these issues as an economist. Apart from other considerations, what this means is that I see health care as something that can be traded and distributed, while health cannot be directly distributed or traded. Consequently, in considering equity I do so in terms of how health care resources 'should' be allocated according to some underlying equity objective.

Equity as a concept

First, what do we mean by equity? It has something to do with fairness and justice, and often has certain aspects of equality attached to or associated with it. But it is not simply – and perhaps not at all – equality of people, but rather equality with respect to certain attributes of people. One of the difficulties is to sort out which attributes are relevant to equity or, more strictly, to this equality.

Getting to the equitable distribution of that 'something' can be done in two ways. First, there is the equitable distribution of the something. The judgement with respect to what is fair is to be made in terms of whether the resultant distribution – what emerges – is fair. This is, in essence, the nature of what is normally called 'distributive justice'. If we are concerned about the distributive justice of health care with respect to health, then we would look to see how health is distributed in a society or community.

A second approach is to adopt the view that it is the mechanisms, rules or procedures involved in deciding on the distribution that need to be judged to be fair. Adopting this stance means that whatever distribution of the something emerges is by definition fair, since it was arrived at through a process deemed to be fair. This second approach is referred to as 'procedural justice'.

The terminology will emerge as important later, but while not quite the same thing, the former is in essence about the fairness of the outcome and the latter about the fairness of the process. These two are not necessarily mutually exclusive but they do represent very different and importantly different ways of viewing equity and fairness.

Another important consideration is that in philosophy there are different ways of viewing equity. There is no single way of doing so. There is likely to be a need to choose between competing philosophical notions or theories of equity.

Underlying these different theories is a still more fundamental issue. Earlier philosophers tended to think that equity could only be viewed from a disinterested or impartial stance. Most frequently quoted in this context is John Rawls' (1971) theory of justice. In order to achieve impartiality, Rawls suggested that individuals should be placed behind a 'veil of ignorance' such that they did not know what their own position in society would be. They were then asked what sort of society they would choose to live in. The society that emerges is one which gives the greatest advantage to the least well off in society. Thus the impartiality here leads to this 'maximising' of the 'minimum' position and it is arrived at through the impartiality created by the veil of ignorance – the so-called maxi-min solution.

More recently (see, for example, Taylor, 1989) philosophers have adopted a somewhat different stance and argued that there is no reason for a just society to be judged solely from an impartial stance. This is partly a reflection of the fact that while Rawls' theory did represent a major breakthrough in thinking about a just society, the Rawlsian solution was not unproblematic. For example while the theory allows for what happens to the least well off, it tells us nothing about other groups in society. In the context of health care it might suggest that the most severely ill get priority, but it does not say to what extent they should get priority. In the context of resource allocation the answer could be: to the extent that that group ceases to be the worst off and another group takes its place. And so on. But that in turn implies that the worst off can be helped and made better off. What if the worst off are suffering from a condition for which the health service can do nothing? And would this not mean that resources would be allocated to a very great extent to saving life at the rescue stage or, more accurately – and an important difference – to *attempting* to save life at that rescue stage? It is perhaps not surprising that Arrow (1974) has suggested that Rawls as applied to health care is likely to end up bankrupting a society.

A further issue, and one that is less often debated, is that Rawls also assumes that individuals behind the veil of ignorance are risk-averse, i.e. they are not prepared to gamble. This means that they will invariably place a high weighting on avoiding being in a very bad position. It follows automatically, given the veil of ignorance and risk aversion, that the Rawlsian 'solution' is bound to be what it is. The terms set by Rawls for examining the problem in fact dictate that a maxi-min solution is the only one possible.

Another question related to Rawls, but not unique to his theory, is that in so far as there clearly are different theories and hence 'solutions' to equity objectives in health care, how do we choose between them? If this is all to be done behind a veil of ignorance, what are the criteria for choosing between theories? Here I would argue that some sort of societal preferences ought to be what decides between competing equity theories and solutions. So my point is that even if we could select equity theories according to some impartial view, we then have to say which is to be preferred. But that seems impossible from behind a veil of ignorance.

But let us assume that somehow there is a uniquely correct solution to the equity objective. That would mean that the question of choosing between alternatives is unnecessary. There is only one. But it is frequently the case that equity and efficiency in health care clash and that achieving greater equity results in less efficiency. What then? What relative weight is to be attached to equity as compared with efficiency?

One way of dealing with this issue, as Culyer (1980) and others have suggested, is to argue that equity as a goal is to be sought irrespective of the cost, and consequently irrespective of the impact on efficiency.

Now this is clearly a *very* strong equity principle. Irrespective of the cost of achieving it, any equity goal chosen is to be pursued and the choice of that equity goal should not be influenced by the cost of achieving it. What it means is that since the cost will be in terms (largely) of health, much suffering and death will occur to allow the goal of equity to be pursued. This might be acceptable, or at least more acceptable, if it were the case that in choosing the equity goal consideration were given to the impact of the different possible choices on efficiency and hence on health. But that is not the position that these writers adopt. Cost is not to be a consideration in choosing an equity goal. (This would be of less concern if these same authors chose some equity goal other than that which they do, which happens to be equality of health. Such an equity goal, as will be discussed below, is likely to be particularly 'costly' in terms of the sacrifice of health necessary for its achievement.)

This issue is important in the context of the impartial choice of an equity goal. If impartiality is to be maintained, then this in effect means that the trade-off between equity and efficiency is deemed not to be relevant in deciding what the equity goal is to be. Such a trade-off involves the exercise of 'partial' – as opposed to impartial – preferences about the weights to be attached to equity as compared with efficiency.

But not to take this into account and not to have some idea of what the health costs of equity might be seems far too strong and far too costly a way of defining equity in health care. However, since this form of thinking is so prevalent in the discussion in principle of equity it cannot be dismissed lightly. It may well be the fact that there is this 'absoluteness' to the principle of equity that has led to a divergence between what is stated as the objective of equity in principle and what actually happens on the ground. Operationally, it is frequently the case, as noted at the beginning of this chapter, that policy objectives as stated in 'official' documents and what is done in practice are quite different. There are important inconsistencies here.

Possible options

There are three possibilities for defining equity in health care. These are equality of health, equality of use of health care and equality of access to health care. There are various variations on these key themes (and I will come to these later) especially when the issue of need is brought in, as in equality of use for equal need. Let me examine these three main contenders in turn.

Equality of health

This concept of equity in health care comes under the category of distributive justice rather than procedural justice. It is concerned with the consequences of policy and judges the goodness of any distribution on the basis of the outcome. As such it has nothing to say directly about the process involved in getting to that distribution. It is a consequentialist view of distribution. It is also a narrow consequentialist view in that the only concern it has is with the consequence health while other consequences are ignored. This would mean, for example, that the distribution of information, except where it had a bearing on the distribution of health, would not be an object of concern for those advocating this equity objective in health care. The idea that a health service might want to promote greater equality in terms of information for its own sake would not be – indeed could not be – encompassed within this definition of equity.

It has been argued (see, for example, Culyer, 1988) that since the objective of health care services is to promote health, the equity goal of health care must be conceived in the same terms, i.e. in terms of equality of health. Such an argument has a certain desirable logic at a policy level, and certainly it makes policy making in some ways simpler if both the efficiency goal of health care and the equity goal can be considered in terms of the single dimension of health. It might, however, be argued that this particular form of consistency is an unnecessary constraint on defining equity in health care.

Again, the World Health Organisation appears to be primarily concerned with health as the equity goal in its targets for Health For All. Indeed, these targets seem to be mainly about equity rather than efficiency, and then in terms of trying to equalise health across not just different groups within a society but also across different societies. Thus the same goals have been put forward for all European countries despite the fact that their starting points are very different in terms of the health of the population and the resources available, in the formal health services and beyond, to do anything about the health problems of the respective countries.

What does equality of health mean? Well presumably the idea would not be equality of health across all age and sex groups; this would seem to be biologically impossible. But within age and sex groups, it means just that, i.e. equal or the same health for all. If no more resources are to be made available to health services to achieve this goal, then presumably to achieve this equal health, some people's health will need to improve and some deteriorate.

A further complication, which was highlighted by the UK Black Report (DHSS, 1980) is that health is affected by all sorts of factors. What health services can do to affect the levels of health of populations or groups within populations may often be quite limited. Yet the goal of health services is often stated as equality of health. There seems yet another logical inconsistency here.

If the goal of health services is equality of health, what happens about these other factors? Are they ignored in the allocation of resources – health service or other – in the pursuit of equality of health? Or are they part of the overall equation in deciding how resources are to be used within the health service to promote equity? This is not clear.

But ignoring these problems – as most writers on this topic seem to do – what of the idea that some individuals' health status will go up and some down? Interestingly, one of the key people advocating health as the goal of equity, Tony Culyer (1991), suggests that equality should only be pursued in an upward direction, i.e. that no one's health should be diminished as part of the process towards achieving equality of health. This suggests that equality of health must be a very long-term goal as the levelling-up process is likely to take generations to have any real impact. Furthermore, for those who are already healthy the chances are that they will get still healthier, even if there were some sort of negative discrimination against them in the allocation of health service resources. So the target level at which health will become equal will tend to be moving upwards anyway.

Of course, it is possible to say that no one's health should decline as part of the process of pursuing equality of health, but this seems unrealistic. How far does a health service go in pursuit of equity to stop individuals' health status declining? The implications in terms of efficiency of such a policy are potentially very great. There is an odd logic to this idea. However, one can see that deliberately to set out to worsen individuals' health status to achieve greater equality of health may be unacceptable.

But are we then not likely to be left with a non-equity policy? If something is efficient, then it should be pursued. Any interference with this will mean that we hold back on the production of health benefits and that thereby someone's health will suffer somewhere whatever their existing level of health. So the idea that no one should be held back means that all that is efficient should be pursued and that therefore any concern for equity which has an adverse effect on efficiency should not be permitted. We then have a 'non-equity' policy!

Let me look at this from a different perspective. What conditions would be required to allow, and indeed justify, an equity goal of equality of health? Not everyone is born with the same health endowment. To attempt to overcome this would presumably require substantial investment in those born with poorer health levels. However, it is clear that this would be a very expensive policy to implement and indeed could not be wholly successful since some of these poorer levels of health with which individuals are born cannot be rectified – at least not with current technology – whatever the level of resources we invest.

If everyone were born with equal health, then a number of conditions would need to apply before this could be maintained throughout life. One would be that each would have the same or similarly healthy lifestyles. There are two factors here. One is that individuals would need to have the same opportunities to have that same lifestyle (which immediately seems problematical as, for example, it is clear that some occupations are more likely to be injurious to health than others). And second, they would need to have the same preferences for these lifestyles. It is difficult to see that those who favoured a sporting life would over time have the same health status as those who favoured reading and little exercise. But then, of course, it would be possible to allocate resources in such a way as to try to compensate those with a tendency to an unhealthy lifestyle. But it is only if individuals have a similar opportunity and exercise it similarly, i.e. have similar preferences for a particular lifestyle, that they will maintain equally healthy lives. (Compensating those with an unhealthy lifestyle leads very likely to a form of moral hazard which will encourage slothfulness, or at least less healthy lifestyles.)

And what of health services? If they are to be used as the vehicle for the pursuit of equality of health, then a number of considerations come into play. Let us assume that individuals do have the same health status to start with. Maintaining this presumably will require that, when faced with some health problem (to which we will assume they are equally susceptible), their reactions will need to be the same, and on three fronts. First, they will need to have the same access to health care. Second, they will need to respond equally to the treatment they receive (or those who are less responsive or more responsive to treatment will require to have positive or negative discrimination). And third, they will need to have the same preferences for both health care and health. They will thus require the same values with respect to health and health care.

In so far as these conditions do not apply there will be a need to discriminate in the treatment of individuals if the goal of equality of health is to be maintained. There seems little that can be done to prevent differences in genetic endowments (in the absence of a programme of genetic engineering). Giving everyone the same chance of the same lifestyle seems very problematical. Some efforts could certainly be made to have more egalitarianism in education by creating more equal opportunities. But even if such a policy were politically acceptable, its success in terms of creating individuals with equal choice sets is unlikely. And even if that did occur, it is quite likely that individuals will choose to exercise their preferences for lifestyles differently. This in turn will have differential effects on their health status.

It is difficult to see how a health service could cope with differential effectiveness across different individuals. It is possible, but almost certainly at the expense of considerable loss of efficiency in the system. Finally, not to allow individuals to have or to exercise different behaviour patterns reflecting different values for health and health care would seem to go against the sorts of principles of autonomy common to most societies, and certainly against the sorts of views on autonomy which most health services would probably espouse.

Equality of health may be possible. Whether it is desirable, given what would be required to achieve it, is something that I will leave the reader to judge. But it does seem to me that it is simply too costly in terms of health and too intrusive in terms of individual values. However, as I indicated before, there is the issue not so much of what is right and wrong but rather what is consistent with a society's values. But then looked at in these terms, i.e. in terms of consistency with a society's values, there would seem to be few societies which would endorse the sorts of values it would be necessary to endorse for equal health to be a desirable and consistent goal for that society.

Of course, it is possible to argue that individuals should be healthy. Health care in this context is a merit good. It might further be argued that information with respect to health and health care is a merit good and that individuals should have an equal chance to choose a healthy lifestyle and to choose health and health care. To argue, however, that health is the merit good, as I would suggest is necessary as a basis for agreeing to equality of health as the equity goal of health care, is not in line with the sorts of values that most societies would endorse.

So why is equal health so popular as an equity goal? I suspect it is for two, simple reasons. First, unthinkingly, what else would it be? After all, health services are about health. It must then be the case that whatever is distributionally relevant must be health. Second, the implications, and indeed the assumptions, of a goal of equal health as the equity objective of health services simply have not been thought through in adequate detail. I do not think I have succeeded in setting out all the necessary assumptions nor all the implications. But I would hope to have provided readers with a sufficient picture to cast doubt about the goal of equity in health care being couched in terms of health. For me the assumptions seem unrealistic and in certain instances draconian and in society's terms unacceptable. The implications at a policy level, especially in terms of the adverse impact on health, are just too great for my values. The reader can decide for him/herself.

Equality of use (for equal need)

In this definition, where use is the relevant dimension, it clearly would not be appropriate to have equal use as the objective irrespective of some other characteristic of the individual such as need or demand for health care. So I will assume here that such a characteristic is taken into consideration.

The distinction between need and demand that is important here is that need is normally seen as being defined according to some third party, usually a medically qualified professional. Demand, on the other hand, is the standard economic concept and is thus based on the preference of the individual.

In most health care systems concerned with equity, need would be the basis of concern rather than demand. If it were demand and equitable choices were to be based on individuals' preferences, then presumably the way to achieve that would be in some way or other to subsidise people so that their willingness to pay for and then demand health care was not a function of their ability to pay. Such subsidisation would allow individuals to decide the extent to which they wanted to consume health care and they could, from what would amount to a 'level playing field' with respect to income, decide how much they wished to purchase. Certainly, many health care systems do operate differential payment systems for co-payment, which at least in part are aimed at overcoming the problems of differential ability to pay arising from different levels of income.

The most common form that this takes is simply that those below a certain level of income or who are in receipt of social security benefits will receive free treatment and do not have to pay the co-payment. Or again, those who are chronically sick or are regular users of a service may get it free or pay for a 'season ticket', which per visit results in a lower payment. Or there may be a ceiling on expenditures on co-payment within a specified period, such as a year. But seldom is it the case that there is an attempt to standardise with respect to ability to pay. Rather, the assumption appears to be that there are those who can afford to pay and those who cannot, and this division is then used to decide where the subsidisation starts and ends.

Beyond that, the more major characteristic with respect to equity is need. Unfortunately, as discussed in Chapter 3, the concept of need is the one which creates the most heat and confusion in the health service lexicon. There seems to be increasing agreement that need is not objective but has to involve someone's value judgements, and that that someone is someone other than the patient. It will thus frequently be the medical practitioner, or it may be the health care system or some part of that system.

There are thus two key ways to define need. One is related to the extent of sickness – the more illness there is in a person or a community the greater is the need for health care. The other is a somewhat more subtle variation on that, where need is defined as a capacity to benefit (Culyer, 1991). So the difference is that the latter will be smaller than the former and different in that some needs under the first definition cannot be dealt with by the health care system and as such there will be no capacity to benefit. Also some conditions will give rise to needs in both cases but the second definition will lead to a smaller need, since not all the problems identified in the first definition can be treated and some residual problems will remain. On both grounds, then, needs are smaller generally under the second definition.

In both there is a need for value judgements. In definition 1, there is a requirement to establish what the problems are and their relative magnitude if they are to be compared and/or aggregated. The emphasis in research on this form of need to date seems to be largely epidemiological, i.e. concerned with assessing the incidence and prevalence of conditions in the community and then talking of the need for services for diabetes, for example, on the basis of the extent of diabetes in the relevant community.

But what of the assessment of needs of different diseases? How are these to be aggregated? And even within the same disease, such as diabetes, how are different degrees of severity to be added together and/or compared? To what extent does the existence of the common cold give rise to need relative to, say, pneumonia? We can probably agree that the former merits a lower ranking of need than the latter – but how much lower? What this emphasises, I think, is that under the first definition for most purposes needs ideally should be measured on a cardinal scale, certainly if we are to use them to decide on the relative weight to be attached to meeting them on grounds of equity. If we are arguing that equity should be measured in terms of equal use for equal need, then for unequal need we require some mechanism of measurement which will allow differential needs to be treated equitably.

There are two types of equity here and an important distinction to be drawn between them. The term 'horizontal equity' is normally used to refer to needs that are the same in some relevant dimension, such as degree of sickness; 'vertical equity' is about meeting different needs differentially. It will be clear that it is normally easier to judge the similarity of different needs than to judge the extent of differences in needs. Yet it is necessary to form both sets of judgements if progress is to be made with the use of this definition.

Clearly, some judgement is needed as to what relative weight is to be attached to different conditions or problems. There seems oddly to be little discussion in the health planning literature on this issue. Yet if need is to be the basis for health care planning and resource allocation – whether in terms of equity or allocative efficiency – then some resolution of the problem of weighting need is required. Bigger may be more needful, but how many more resources should be allocated to that greater need, and on what basis?

One way of doing this is to say that needs are to be based on health losses, with the extent of need to be measured by the loss in health to which the condition gives rise. That requires a measure of health loss which might, for example, be QALYs lost. Certainly, some such measure is needed with this first definition.

The second definition leads in practice to still greater problems in at least some respects. Certainly value judgements are again required with respect to the extent of needs and how they are to be added together. Now a further judgement is needed, which is about whether and to what extent there can be a benefit for the sufferers of different conditions. And who is to form the judgement about capacity to benefit? There are two aspects to this. First, there is the issue of benefit. What does that word mean, how is the benefit to be measured and by whom? Presumably, again, we are talking about benefit in terms of health gains, although there seems no reason to exclude other types of benefit such as information. Normally we would argue that the only person who can judge the benefit of health gains is the patient concerned if we genuinely mean benefit in utility terms. When Culyer (1991), for example, writes of capacity to benefit, he is not clear as to whether he means the benefit as assessed by the individual or benefit as assessed by a third party, such as a medical doctor. It seems that he means assessed by a third party.

Certainly when it comes to the issue of *capacity* to benefit, capacity here would presumably be judged by an expert third party. The individual is unlikely to be in a position to form that judgement. But again there are value judgements here which are not present under the first definition. The extent to which someone may benefit from treatment does involve technical judgements, but it also involves value judgements when that capacity to benefit idea is to be applied to more than one condition at a time or to more than one level of severity even within the same condition.

I am not going to attempt to resolve these issues here. I would simply point to the fact that immediately we get into discussions of need in the context of how equity is to be handled, then it is not just the definition of equity with respect to, say, use versus health that becomes complex but also the definition of need. There remain beyond that difficulties with how that definition can be effected and with deciding on the basis of whose value judgements this is to be done. This is an area where we need much more thought and discussion in health policy circles. There is a paucity of thought here, which is odd given the central importance attached to the concept in much of recent health care planning.

In choosing between need as a reflection of the size of a problem and need as the potential within the problem to produce benefit, there is a good argument for adopting the capacity to benefit definition, If resources are to be allocated equitably, then to do so on the basis of the potential for production of benefit would seem a more reasonable way to go than simply *pro rata* with the size of the problems. However, that leaves a number of difficulties, particularly with respect to values.

It also leaves an issue that seems not to have been addressed in the literature at all. It is quite likely that for the majority of starting points that we might be dealing with, capacity to benefit will be subject to diminishing returns. In other words, as the capacity to benefit declines, so it will become increasingly more costly to get a further increase in benefit. This means that any allocation of resources which is made on the basis of need – of capacity to benefit – ought to reflect this diminishing marginal benefit effect. Yet I am not aware that those formulae, such as RAWP (DHSS, 1976), which do attempt to allocate resources equitably according to some needs-based formula, allow for this. This is almost certainly because these formulae are based on the first definition of need and not on the second. As such they do not need to reflect this consideration of diminishing returns since they allocate simply on the basis of the size of the problem and not the prospects of benefit from intervention.

What, then, of the more basic aspect of equity here, i.e. the notion of equality of use? It is a common definition among researchers and, for example, is the basis of much of the work by van Doorslaer *et al.* (1993) in their mammoth study of equity in health care in the European Common Market.

Use here equals actual consumption, and actual consumption is a function not just of demand (or need) but also of supply. Individuals may demand but not get because, for example, the price is too high or there is some deficiency in supply. Patients may be deemed to be in need, but again not actually receive because there are higher priority cases who force them out; or at best they have to wait. So consumption and use are not the same as demand or need.

A more reasoned case, perhaps rather oddly, can be made for use being equated with supply. This will occur where there is excess demand or excess need so that whatever is supplied will be used. Thus assuming that there is greater need for services than are supplied, then the equity approach which embraces equal use for equal need will be incorporated in an approach which adopts the position of *supplying* services *pro rata* with need. But this in turn requires that need and demand are the same, otherwise the fact that capacity to benefit as assessed by experts is greater than supply will not necessarily mean that what patients demand is the same as their capacity to benefit.

Where this is not the case then they may 'underuse' services, and in turn supply and use will not be the same.

Thus use can be equated with supply where there is excess need and where need rather than demand is the basis of the way in which patients actually make use of health services. However, if patients' preferences are important in using health services, i.e. if their use is based on their demands to at least some extent, then the equation of supply with use will not follow.

This leads us on to what seems a fundamental issue on this definition of equity. It would appear to ignore the possibility that individuals will have demands for health care and that the exercise of their preferences with respect to the use of services might lead to some differences in the way in which services are used as compared with what would occur if the service use were based solely on need.

This is an issue of some moment in the debate about the definition of equity, as I have suggested elsewhere (Mooney *et al.*, 1991). However, Culyer *et al.* (1992) have responded by suggesting that 'policy makers would want to know the reasons for the differing demand curves before they make their judgement (as to whether these variations in demand are of no consequence)'.

Grossmann and Leeder (1991) also question whether we cannot (or should not) be more ambitious than to settle for access as the dimension of equity. They ask: 'Is a vigorous and physically accessible health care sector our vision, or will we let ourselves be more ambitious than that?'

Now clearly there are very different points of view here. My concern is not with some normative view of what the goal of equity should be, and both Culyer *et al.* and Grossman and Leeder seem to be moving towards a normative view. But normatively or positively, where I think the difference lies between the two opposing points of view is in the role of demand in a needs-based service.

My own view is that even in a needs-based service, demand remains relevant. What services are available may well be needs based and once individuals enter the service their use may be heavily influenced by their medical practitioner's assessment of their need. But entering the service – especially visits to the GP as the start of use of the service for a particular episode of care – will be largely demand-based.

'Compliance', which is about the relationship between need and demand after the first contact, is frequently not perfect. This would seem to provide evidence that need and demand do diverge.

But there remains the issue of whether it is 'legitimate' that they diverge, or whether such divergences should be tolerated, or even where they exist attempts made to reduce or eliminate them. The issue seems very clear cut at the level of the first contact. This, in most instances, has to be demand based. For subsequent contacts it is a very patronising or at best paternalistic attitude not to allow individuals to choose whether to accept the advice of their GPs or their medical practitioners more generally. The implication too is that doctors are perfect agents for their patients with respect not just to their patients' health but to their patients' utility more generally. That seems unlikely. Consequently, unless one does take a very optimistic view of the perfection of agency and one believes in a very paternalistic health service, then it seems desirable to allow demand – essentially patients' varying preferences – to continue to be relevant in the consumption of health services. (For more debate about agency, see Chapter 6.)

In the context not just of equity but also with respect to the issue of what is in the patient's utility function and also what it is with respect to the patient's welfare that the perfect agent is trying to maximise or should be trying to maximise, one important point to note is the following. A definition of equity, which assumes that the goal is equal use for equal need, is ignoring not just variations in individuals' preferences for health but variations in individuals' preferences for health care. Yet the *process* of consumption of health services may well involve varying utility or disutility for different individuals. Some, for example, may have more fear of dentists than others. Yet equal use as a criterion for equity would seem intent on not allowing such variations to be taken into account in devising equitable health care policies.

So the advocates of equal use as the basis for equity in health care are arguing either that all should or that all do value health equally, and further that they also value the process of consuming health care equally. Neither of these assumptions would seem to stand up to serious examination. Consequently I would suggest that equal use for equal need as a criterion for equity in health care is seriously flawed and ill-conceptualised.

It may be that those who advocate equal use for equal need are in fact seeing this as purely instrumental in pursuit of the goal of equal health. The question then – ignoring the other problems I have identified above – is: would equal use for equal need lead to equal health?

Equal health is about eliminating inequalities in health. It presumably is about discriminating between people who have different needs in such a way as to move them closer to equal health and hence equal needs, and eventually eliminate differences in health states. There are a number of steps involved in this process and it is worth looking at them in a little detail in the context of equal use being instrumental as a route to equal health.

The first point to note is that equal use for equal need is a form of horizontal equity. Equals (in terms of need) should be treated equally. Now as indicated above, if advocates of equal use for equal need see such a policy as instrumental in the pursuit of the 'final' goal of equal health, then to discriminate between those with equal needs might well increase health inequalities. However, this is not necessarily the case. Individuals with the same need – in terms of capacity to benefit – may not be equally responsive to treatment. Consequently, to give them equal treatment will not maintain their health status at the same level.

The second point is perhaps still more fundamental. If a policy is aimed at eliminating differences in health status through equality of use, then it must say something about how reductions in differentials in health status are to be brought about, and the extent to which use is to be unequal *vis-à-vis* variations in need to allow that to occur. Yet it is clear that equal use for equal need is an equity policy which is about horizontal equity and says nothing in itself about differential use for differential need. As a criterion of equity, it cannot be defended with respect to being instrumental in the pursuit of equality of health because such a policy would need to provide guidance on the reduction or elimination of differences in health status through differential need. And equal use for equal need does not provide this guidance. Further, unless patients are equally responsive to treatment when they have the same needs and (returning to what was said above) have the same values for health and for health care consumption, then a policy of equal use for equal need will lead to potentially *wider* differentials in health status.

In essence, therefore, whether equal use for equal need is seen as an equity goal in its own right or as instrumental in the pursuit of equal health, it does not seem to stand up to serious examination. As a goal in its own right, it has major value problems and leaves health care as a merit good, since it denies the relevance of individuals' values in the consumption of health care. As instrumental in the pursuit of equal health, it might lead to increasing rather than decreasing differences in health status, depending on how serious and how prevalent the issue of differential responsiveness to treatment is across different patients with the same needs. And it provides no guidance with respect to what to do about discriminating between different needs. How different should use be to achieve reductions in, and eventually eliminate, differences in health states? This question, which is critical to the achievement of equal health, is not addressed by the equal use for equal need approach to equity.

Equality of access (for equal need)

There are problems in defining the word 'access' in the context of health care which make any definition of equity that is dependent on access difficult. Yet it seems to be the most commonly found definition of equity in policy documents (Donaldson and Gerard, 1993).

There are two key concepts of equality of access. In one the opportunity cost is the same and in the other the welfare cost is the same. (Presumably there is also a possibility of some mix of the two.) The opportunity cost one (which I tend to think is both the more likely and the more useful in policy terms) states that two individuals have equal access if the costs to them in using the service – in terms of opportunities forgone – are valued the same. Note that this does not mean that they are necessarily the same in the sense of being, say, 'physically' the same, e.g. each lives the same distance from the GP's surgery. And even if the 'physical' opportunity cost – *what* is forgone (as opposed to the *benefit* forgone, which clearly has to have a value attached to it) – is the same, it does not follow that the cost to the two individuals is the same. For example, if each gives up a round of golf to visit an outpatient department and that is, to each, the next best use of their time, the value they each attach to the forgone game need not be the same. And of course, the time given up may well have different 'physical' opportunity costs. So the idea of equality of access being defined in terms of equality of opportunity cost is not without difficulties in practice. (Indeed, as I indicate in more detail below, there is a strong case for more research into just how one can best identify opportunity costs in this context, and in turn how these can be measured and equated across different individuals.)

With respect to the 'welfare loss' concept of cost, what this means is that for access to be the same, the disutility of the involvement in the treatment is the same for the two individuals. This would include, for example, the loss in utility to an individual female patient who had a preference for a female gynaecologist rather than a male gynaecologist but the hospital only had male gynaecologists. Or it would mean in practice trying somehow to allow the patient who was particularly fearful of operations to be compensated for this in some way such that his or her loss of utility in facing an operation was the same as those of less fearful patients.

While I would not want to suggest that this is not a legitimate way to see access, in practice I think it is unhelpful and potentially confusing. And it is certainly difficult to bring about – more so than the opportunity cost definition. Fortunately too, I think it is unnecessary to go down this welfare loss road in defining access, especially once one allows the notion of process utility and perhaps also other aspects of outcome utility (other than health, that is) to come legitimately into the patient's utility function.

This is because once the process utility of being treated is included, then it can be placed on the 'demand side' of the equation and access can be kept, as I tend to think is desirable, as a wholly supply-side phenomenon. Thus the question arises about equal access to what and how, once having gained access, people maximise their utility. But that becomes a 'post-access' issue.

One of the particular advantages of this approach is that it avoids the adoption of an elitist stance to health and to health care. The issue of access being wholly supply-side-based means that what is being provided is an equal availability, and equal opportunity to use the service, but not equality of use. Thus equal access still allows individuals, should they so wish, to express their preferences for consuming health care or not according to their own preferences for health and for health care.

It is likely, however, that equal access will be tied to the idea of need and that the goal will be equal access for equal need. This is less problematical than for equal use for equal need in that it does not require people to use health care at a particular level commensurate with their level of need as does the equal use definition. This seems a major difference, and in terms of the sorts of values that I would want to see apply in health care more realistic and appropriate. Clearly, there is scope for different values here. While I can see that access may be something that many can agree on in the sense of wanting equal access for all, I find it difficult to see that there would be the same agreement in the community for an equity goal which was equal use for equal need and which denied individuals the right to exercise their own preferences for health and for health care. But of course – and fortunately! – this is an empirically verifiable issue.

There is also a level at which equal access does not have to be tied to need, and in a way which is different from use. This is at the most general level of the health care process as a system. At any point in time most of the population will not be consuming health care, but none the less in terms of the choice of a system of health care may well favour one which provides equal access for all, should they require health care. In this very general sense all are more or less equally at risk of future problems and as such need is less important. Of course, there are situations where it will be desirable to tie access to need, for example, in setting up some way of allocating funds for health care geographically and where to maintain the idea of equality of access, say, for diabetics or for those with heart problems or whatever, we would want to take some account of the needs in different populations.

Indeed, this is probably the only situation in which there is a case for measuring total needs in any population. (See the discussion of total needs assessment in Chapter 3.)

Again, as with use, it is possible to argue that access is not the goal and is only instrumental, and that the goal remains equal health. However, the links from access to health are even more tortuous than the links from use to health (as discussed above). Consequently, I do not think it is necessary to demonstrate that for those favouring access as the equity goal it is more than just instrumental. (I need to be quite clear here: the issue is not whether access is instrumental but whether it is *solely* instrumental and not valued at least in part for itself.)

Why, then, would access *per se* have value in itself? Certainly those who are consequentialists, and in particular narrow consequentialists (and who restrict relevant consequences to health), will have difficulties in accepting the notion that there could be value in the process of making access available equally to different groups in a society. They will have further difficulties perhaps in abandoning the welfare loss definition of access as, being consequentialists, they will not be able to incorporate the process utility into the demand side of the equation.

The answer here would seem to be very simple. Individuals may prefer a health care system which provides equal access for all. They may think that this is fairer. They prefer a society which is fairer to one that is less fair. The particular nature of health and ill-health is such that, as Tobin (1970) has indicated, health is a special case when it comes to egalitarian feelings. These may be present in certain other aspects of a society. Indeed, where this feeling is strong with respect to health care, it may well be that it is also present with respect to at least some other aspects of life in that society. This would seem to be the case, for example, in much of Scandinavia where equity in health care does seem to be highly valued and where this is part of a wider concern in these societies for equity more generally, often described under the heading of 'solidarity'.

It is this phenomenon of valuing equity or going even further and participating in creating a fairer society that lies behind the notion of Margolis (1982) of what he describes as 'doing our fair share', or more formally 'participation utility'. Here Margolis assumes that individuals get utility from making their own contribution to the society, or the community, or the group to which they belong, and of which they are a member.

The idea is also reflected at a policy level in the following comment from Nye Bevan, the founder of the NHS in the United Kingdom:

> No society can legitimately call itself civilised if a sick person is denied medical aid because of lack of means . . . .. Society becomes more

wholesome, more serene, and spiritually healthier, if it knows that its
citizens have at the back of their consciousness the knowledge that not only
themselves, but all their fellows, have access, when ill, to the best that
medical skill can provide. (in Foot, 1975)

Note here that what Bevan is writing about is access, and that he sees
this as leading in health care to a more serene society.

There seems not much more to add about access, and while I am
sure that my bias is clear with respect to which of the three dimensions
– health, use or access – is and should be the goal of equity, I do have
difficulties in seeing the merits of health or use. But I also accept that
there are clear value judgements involved in making the choice and
not all readers will agree with my value judgements.

As a final note to this debate, I think a refinement of access as the
relevant dimension of equity may be appropriate. While I reject use of
health care and health because they have merit good or merit want
connotations, I think there may be a case for not allowing individuals
to be more ignorant than necessary about their health and about
prospects for improving their health through health care. Thus there
may be a case for altering the equal access definition to make it equally
informed access. If individuals have equal access and then have
different use because they are differentially informed about their
health despite their needs being the same and differentially informed
about the prospects for improving their health as a result of actually
consuming health care, then I do wonder whether this knowledge
difference ought not to be corrected or at least addressed. In other
words, I do not want health care to be a merit good but it may be that
information about health and about health care ought to be treated as
a merit good.

Concluding comments

I hope that this chapter will have given the reader some basis for
thinking further about equity in health care and that you will be
stimulated to think more about some of the issues that I have raised. I
tend to think that equity is a rather complex phenomenon. It may be,
however, that having thought quite a lot about it in recent years I am
making it unnecessarily complex. I hope that is true, but I am
doubtful. Certainly I am struck by two things about equity in health
care: it is an important aspect or goal of most health care systems; and
second, there seems to be continuing confusion about what it is about
and how it is to be defined (although this confusion seems greater in
the minds of researchers than it is in the minds of policy makers).

There is plenty of scope for further research on the topic and for multidisciplinary work to be done. (In reading about equity, and I am as guilty as anyone else in this respect, I am fascinated to note how economists quote other economists when writing on the topic, philosophers quote philosophers, and so on. Yet here surely, of all the topics touched on in this book, is the one where cross-disciplinary fertilisation is likely to prove most useful.)

Perhaps there is a growing acceptance that access is an important dimension of equity whether it is solely instrumental or not. That suggests that, while defining access is difficult, the sort of working definition I have proposed may be enough to let us get on to look at the issue of measurement.

As long as researchers go on measuring the wrong things – health and use of health care – which is what they seem intent on doing (see, for example, Wagstaff *et al.*, 1991), then the cause of equity in policy circles will not be advanced. We need to measure the right thing, and I am clear that the right thing is access, even if I am less than certain that the definition – equal opportunity cost of use – is as good as it might be. I am convinced, however, that it is this issue that is most important. Research on health services with respect to equity must be able to measure variations in access so that this variable, i.e. access, can be monitored. That is the key issue.

For those readers who do not share my enthusiasm for access as the dimension of equity, perhaps the key target for research ought to be to try to establish what the community believes the definition of equity ought to be, or perhaps simply is. Unless one adopts the view – as some do – that any definition of equity has to be made from an impartial stance, then the resolution of how to define equity in health care is again simple. We need to go out and ask people what it is. Maybe that is the even more fundamental research issue for the next year or two.

References

Arrow, K. J. (1974) Gifts and exchanges. *Philosophy and Public Affairs*, 1, 343–62.
Birch, S. and Abelson, J. (1992) Is reasonable access what we want? McMaster University Centre for Health Economics and Policy Analysis, Hamilton.
Culyer, A. J. (1980) *The Political Economy of Social Policy*. Martin Robertson, Oxford.
Culyer, A. J. (1988) Inequalities of health services is, in general, desirable. In D. G. Green (ed.) *Acceptable Inequalities? Essays in the Pursuit of Equality in Health Care*. IEA, London.

Culyer, A. J. (1991) Equity in health care policy. Paper prepared for the Ontario Premier's Council on Health, Well-Being and Social Justice. University of Toronto, Toronto.

Culyer, A. J., van Doorslaer, E. and Wagstaff, A. (1992) Comment on: *Utilisation as a Measure of Equity* by Mooney *et al. Journal of Health Economics*, **11**, 93–8.

DHSS (1976) *Report of the Resource Allocation Working Party* (RAWP). HMSO, London.

DHSS (1980) *Inequalities in Health* (The Black Report). DHSS, London.

Donaldson, C. and Gerard, K. (1993) *Economics of Health Care Financing*. Macmillan, London.

van Doorslaer, E., Wagstaff, A. and Rutten, F. (eds) (1993) *Equity in the Finance and Delivery of Health Care. An International Perspective.* Oxford Medical Publications, Oxford.

Foot, M. (1975) *Aneurin Bevan, 1945–1960*. Paladin, London.

Grossman, J. and Leeder, S. R. (1991) A din of inequity. *Australian Journal of Public Health*, **15**, 2–4.

Margolis, H. (1982) *Selfishness, Altruism and Rationality*. Cambridge University Press, Cambridge.

Mooney, G., Hall, J., Donaldson, C. and Gerard, K. (1991) Utilisation as a measure of equity: weighing heat? *Journal of Health Economics*, **10**, 4, 383–476.

Rawls, J. (1971) *A Theory of Justice*. Harvard University Press, Cambridge, Mass.

Taylor, C. (1989) *Sources of the Self: The making of modern identity*. Harvard University Press, Cambridge, Mass.

Tobin, J. (1970) Limiting the domain of inequality. *Journal of Law and Economics*, **13**, 263–77.

Wagstaff, A., van Doorslaer, E. and Pace, P. (1991) On the measurement of horizontal inequity in the delivery of health care. *Journal of Health Economics*, **10**, 169–206.

6

Agency in health care

Introduction

It is one of the central tenets of health economics that health care is different. What is meant by this? In economic terms it is an attempt to establish that, as compared with other goods and services which may be provided in an efficient way through the private market, health care is such that such markets are unlikely to be the best way to 'buy and sell' this particular commodity.

Such a view seems unexceptionable, at least to this economist. However, it is important to recognise that not all economists would share it. Especially in the United States there are many economists who still hold to the view that health care can be successfully (i.e. efficiently) provided in the private market. (There are few who would argue so readily that it can be provided equitably on the private market but that is only a problem if equity is a goal of health care. Normally private health care would seem not to subscribe to equity as an appropriate goal for a health care system.)

However, the view expressed here is that health care creates very real problems for the private individual, as a consumer, with respect to information. For private markets to work well a number of features are required. Included in these, and particularly relevant to the question of health care, is that the consumers have perfect information. Now while it is certainly the case that there are few markets where consumer information is perfect, the imperfections of information for the consumer in the health care market are very great indeed. The consumer is unlikely to have good information about her own health state, what treatments are available, what the effectiveness of treatments is likely to be and what the cost of the treatments will be. Additionally, there may be problems for the consumer in translating effectiveness in terms of health into 'utility'. (For more on utility and utility functions, see Chapters 1 and 2.) Thus while it is often assumed in the literature in health economics that the consumer is the only one who can make the link between health status changes and utility gains and losses, there is perhaps a need to recognise that while true there are problems for the consumer in performing this linkage. (This issue will be returned to below.)

One feature of the market which is perhaps understated in considerations of the debate about the relevance of the market to the provision of health care is that very often the consumer will be aware of her own deficiencies with respect to making rational choices. There are many areas of life where we are less than fully informed but where none the less we make the choices. We do so sometimes believing that we are well informed, or at least that we are sufficiently well informed to do so. The question of 'sufficiently' may be important here.

Making the wrong choices in some areas of life – normal market decisions about purchasing electrical goods, cars, even houses – can lead to problems. They are unlikely, however, to be of the same magnitude on average as getting choices wrong with health care purchases. Further, what the health care market has that many other markets do not is a group of highly trained professionals operating according to an ethical code which pushes them (or constrains them, depending on one's viewpoint) to do the best they can for their patients. Thus in health care the patient is central and the idea is that the doctor puts the patient before self in making decisions about patient care.

There is thus the idea (Evans, 1984) of the agent (doctor) acting on behalf of the uncertain and ill-informed patient (principal). The patient is ill informed and knows it. The doctor is better informed and both she and the patient know it. The patient is then 'in the doctor's hands' with respect to what health care to demand. This 'agency relationship' is absolutely central to health care and certainly to health economics. Yet the extent to which it is understood seems more limited than it ought to be given its central role in health care (Mooney and Ryan, 1993). Further, there is a lack of understanding on the part of the profession as to what their legitimate role is with respect to agency, and at least disagreement within the profession as to what the agency role's object ought to be. Is the doctor trying to maximise the patient's health or to maximise patient utility, where it is assumed that utility includes health but also possibly other considerations? Put in another way, is the doctor trying to make the patient only healthier, or does some wider concern with happiness come into the picture – a happiness which includes health but other matters as well? Or again, seen more broadly, is the doctor trying to maximise on behalf of the group of patients for whom she is – say, as a GP – responsible? Or wider still, is the doctor an agent for society, trying to use the resources at her disposal in the most efficient or the most equitable way possible from the point of view of society?

In this chapter I want to consider this agency role. I do not think that the reader will find answers to all these questions. However, in terms of the future directions of health care policy there is a need for more debate and, through that, more understanding of the agency relationship in health care. If health policy is to work in the sense of promoting efficiency and equity in health care, then this cannot be achieved without an appropriate interaction between patients and their doctors within the system. But what is appropriate, and how can health policy best address the question of how to achieve that appropriate interaction?

I have devoted much of a separate chapter to the issue of competition in health care (see Chapter 10). However, this chapter has a bearing on that. At a time when several health care systems are introducing, or are thinking of introducing, greater competition, and where privatisation remains on the agenda of policy makers in health care, the role of financing in affecting the agency role needs examination. There is no doubt that different financing arrangements can provide different forms of incentives and incentive structures on the actors in health care. Not all of these structures will promote greater efficiency, and certainly not all will promote equity. These issues will also be considered within this chapter.

In the next section I shall consider a little more the question: why agency in health care?, as that is fundamental to all that follows. Next I shall examine what sort of role we might ideally want from our doctors, seen from the standpoints of the individual patient, of the patients of the doctor and of society more generally. Thereafter I will set out some of the ideas on agency which are current in health economics and finally try to assess where agency has got to in health care and what we might best do to get doctors to act as 'perfect agents' – indeed, what that term would ideally mean.

Why agency?

Agency in economics more generally arises because of the fact that there are situations in which the potential consumer recognises that he or she is not well equipped to make rational, informed consumption decisions. She then decides to rely on someone acting on her behalf who is an expert or at least better informed. The potential consumer recognises that she has a better chance of maximising utility with such assistance. The agent is then 'employed' to assist the 'principal'. In doing so, there very often has to be some careful working out of the fees and fee structure needed to try to get the agent to act in the consumer's best interests, while recognising at the same time that the agent is also trying to maximise her utility. (For more detail of the principal–agent relationship in economics more generally, see for example MacDonald, 1984; Arrow, 1986.)

The situation in health care is similar but with one important distinction from this standard approach. This is that it is argued that there is not complete independence of the consumer's and the supplier's utility functions in the case of health care. The doctor gains utility from helping a patient to get better, for example, so that the patient's health is an argument not just in the patient's utility function but also in the doctor's utility function. And of course, there may be other arguments in the patient's utility function that are common to the doctor's utility function (and just which these might be is another important aspect of the discussion of what constitutes the perfect agent).

It will readily be apparent that the situation in health care fits this general picture rather well. We have a 'consumer', the patient, who is ill informed and a doctor who is able to act as the more informed agent on behalf of the patient. The patient is ill informed on a number of levels but not necessarily equally ill informed at all levels. (Attending a GP for a first visit is a rather different consumption decision from being admitted to a coronary care unit.)

The types of information that the patient may lack will include: (1) information about her health status; (2) information about the available treatments; and (3) information about the effectiveness of treatment. As indicated above, it is also likely that while it is normally assumed it is the patient who makes the link between changed health status and utility, there is a clear sense in which in some circumstances the doctor will assist in this process as well. But of course, it will *have* to be the case in many instances that the patient does make the link between health and utility. Agency arises because of the gap in information between the patient and the doctor.

While this is unexceptionable, and I think very clear, what is less often discussed and considered is just how this information gap exists and whether the agency role is constant across the different forms of information deficiency. It is therefore worth considering each of the above in turn although, while potentially separable, points 2 and 3 are sufficiently closely related to be taken together.

Health status

When a patient first attends the doctor, it will frequently be the case that she does so because of some particular symptom which she may or may not have experienced before. This can range from a very specific concern where the patient is rather well informed because she has had the same symptom before and the doctor was able to identify the problem previously – something like influenza would be a case in point. Here the patient is clear about what is wrong and probably also rather clear about what should be done about it. (Or at least there will be some fairly clear expectations based on previous experience.)

Here the agency role of the doctor is minimal, especially if the doctor is already familiar with the patient and knows her medical history. The circumstances are rather similar to more 'normal' market transactions. Even here, however, it is possible that agency applies in that the symptoms may well not be identical or they may be recurring sufficiently frequently for the patient to think that something else or something more serious is wrong. So even at this minimalist level aspects of agency may still be present.

Where the symptoms have not been experienced before, or are very unusual, or anxiety-creating in some way or other, then agency will more readily apply. The patient not only wants to know (normally) what is wrong but also whether it is likely to prove serious or whether it is a simple condition that, with no or minimal treatment, will sort itself out. Here much of the role of the agent is not just about information with respect to diagnosing what is wrong, but also giving information to the patient in such a way that the patient understands it and is not unnecessarily worried by the process of diagnosing and informing. So here the agency role is not just about the diagnosis so that something can be done in terms of treatment. Already the doctor is potentially taking account of other possible arguments in the patient's utility function.

When a patient is referred further in the system or is involved in a return visit to a GP, then the lack of information about health status is likely to lead to a higher level of anxiety. Thus while the importance of getting a diagnosis – and getting it right – increases with this later contact, it is likely to be the case that the issue of the relief of anxiety will also increase in importance.

Treatments available and their effectiveness

When it comes to indicating to the poorly informed patient what treatments might be considered and their effectiveness, how this is done may well depend very much on the extent to which the doctor wants to inform the patient and the extent to which the patient wants to be informed. Doctors seem to differ in their views about what it is that patients want from them with respect to choice of treatments. Some will argue that their task is to tell the patient what treatment they should have, i.e. it is for the doctor to consider what the range of possible treatments is, weigh up their effectiveness in the particular circumstances of this patient, and in essence decide on behalf of the patient what the best course of action is. This paternalistic role means that the patient's attitude is not considered relevant when deciding what is the best treatment, and indeed the doctor may also believe that it will worry the patient unnecessarily to get the patient sufficiently informed to make the decision, or that the patient will suffer as a result of having to make the decision.

The doctor may then take this line if she believes that (1) it is her 'responsibility' to propose what she thinks is best for the patient; (2) the patient does not want to be informed; (3) the patient, even if she wants to be informed, will in fact suffer as a result of that information and therefore it is better withheld; (4) the doctor considers that even if informed, the patient will not want to make the decision so she (the doctor) may as well get on with it; or (5) even if the patient wants to be informed and make the decision, the suffering to the patient of making the decision will not be justified and certainly unnecessary so it is better just for the doctor to get on with it.

I have chosen to spell out these options as I think it is important to do so in trying to assess the role of the agent. Whatever that role is, it is likely that not all doctors will agree as to how it is performed 'perfectly' and not all patients will agree either as to how it is performed 'perfectly'. In particular there may well be disagreement among the doctors and the patients on what is the maximand, i.e. what it is that doctors are trying to maximise on behalf of the patients.

A further feature which may be important at this level, especially with respect to the effectiveness of treatments, is that doctors may be uncertain as to how effective different treatments might be. This uncertainty may be a feature of the particular treatment concerned, i.e. there is a genuine lack of knowledge about the effectiveness of a particular treatment for this class of patients. It may also be that the doctor has good information about the effectiveness of the treatment for the appropriate class of patients but is uncertain about the specific effectiveness, given a particular patient and her specific condition and symptoms. Yet again the doctor may be uncertain because she lacks knowledge that does exist, i.e. she is not familiar with the relevant literature which does exist and which, if she knew of it, would reduce or eliminate her uncertainty, at least from this particular source.

Imperfections of knowledge, leading to uncertainty on the part of the doctor, may result in different reactions from the doctor. These reactions may in turn trigger different reactions from the patient. The doctor may openly admit her ignorance or try to cover it up, the likelihood of such reactions probably varying from doctor to doctor. So that uncertainty and its type (of those listed above) may affect the behaviour of the doctor in dealing with the patient and hence the workings of the agency relationship.

These considerations draw us into the debate about precisely what it is that the agency relationship is about. The question of uncertainty, and precisely how doctors cope with it, is less well researched than might have been expected. Yet is it likely that uncertainty is important in both the doctor's utility function and the patient's utility function and hence in agency. At the same time it is unlikely that patients and doctors view uncertainty in the same way, especially when it comes to the issue of who bears the responsibility for the decision making and hence coping with uncertainty.

On the link between changes in health status and utility, while – as indicated above – it is the patient who has to make this link, at the time that a decision is made with respect to, say, choice of treatment, the patient may not be well placed to make this choice. While the doctor might want to restrict her function to explaining what is involved in a particular operation, the chances of success and what success means in terms, say, of physical functioning, the expected physical functioning may be beyond the patient's comprehension. The patient may then look to the doctor for help in *ex ante* making the link between that health status expected and expected utility from that health status. Certainly *ex post* it will be the patient who gets the realised utility, but that is *ex post* and as such is no longer relevant to the decision. There is thus a case for looking at how doctors as agents react to this issue of how patients cope *ex ante* with the health to utility link. (And of course, if there are other arguments in the patient's utility function, then the same considerations may apply to them. However, these are less likely to be ones where the gap between doctor and patient in terms of information and ability to make the appropriate judgements will be as large as it is in the case of health *per se* or go in the same direction. The sorts of issue here will relate to, say, decision making and information.)

The question of the nature of the gaps in information between doctor and patient clearly matters in trying to sort out just how agency works and how it might work better. Unless this is understood, it is unlikely that the goal of a perfect agent will be achieved or even approximated. Just what the perfect agent might look like is important and it is to that that we now turn.

Perfect agency

While there is little agreement in the literature (as I will discuss in the next section) as to what constitutes perfect agency, here I want to put forward my own views on what that might constitute. At the same time I will discuss just how such perfection might be achieved, or at least approached. I shall do so under two headings: first, agency which is perfect from the standpoint of the doctor's patients; and second, agency which is perfect from the standpoint of society as a whole. It would in principle be possible to distinguish in the first case between the individual patient and the patients of a doctor as a group but the idea of the 'index' patient getting unrestricted or unconstrained treatment based on the ethical principle that the doctor must do the best she can for the patient, irrespective of what else the doctor might be doing, is not an economic issue since it denies the scarcity of resources. It is also not related to the real world in which doctors and patients have to operate.

It is worth noting in passing, however, that this unreal world can sometimes be the one that doctors use to try to support their ethical stances – and especially to try to fight off the ideas of economics intruding on their ethical world. Certainly, such a world is likely to be one in which economics has no place to intrude, but since it is an unreal world and one that cannot exist, then to exclude economics from it is not problematical. What can be is if doctors, patients or anyone else are confused about that world as compared to the real world of scarcity, and where choice between patients has to be made. That is potentially dangerous and the distinction here between myth and reality has to be kept very clear at all times.

In the first case, the perfect agent will be one who succeeds, given certain constraints such as resource constraints, in maximising her patients' utility. The first point to note here is that, given the notion of constraints – and especially resource constraints – and the notion of utility maximisation, I think it is legitimate to claim that this is at least in part an economic issue. There is choice under a constrained budget and utility is to be maximised within that.

What will be the arguments in the patient's utility function? I think it is safe to assume that health will normally be there and in some cases will not just dominate but also monopolise the utility function. But other arguments will be present at least in certain instances. The most likely candidates for inclusion here will be information (and as indicated above, this can be of various types); involvement in the decision-making process (or avoidance of such involvement); and various aspects of the process of decision making and treatment. The process aspects will include the dignity and respect shown to the patient by the professional staff generally and not just by the doctors; and the administrative functioning of the service. This can cover whether the receptionist smiles, to an explicit caring attitude on the part of the staff generally, all the way through to the sorts of patient satisfaction issues that are increasingly being monitored in patient contacts with the service – punctuality of staff, politeness, whether the waiting areas are clean and tidy, etc. Not all of these will come into the realm of influence of the medical doctor. It is on those which do that I will concentrate here.

I discuss at greater length in Chapter 11 what patients want from their health service and what these arguments might be. However, the key points to make here are, first, that I would judge that it is very likely that the arguments will extend beyond health; second, that in order to determine this research must be done on patients' wishes; and third, that the medical profession could be better trained to find out what patients want and thereafter change their behaviour accordingly to try to maximise their patients' utility. I am clear that the vast majority of doctors faced with the question 'what are you trying to maximise on behalf of your patients?' would respond by saying 'their health'. It may be that that is the right thing for them to be doing, but I doubt it. Certainly I think there is a strong case for trying to find out more about this issue. Of course, it will be complicated by the fact that not all patients will agree what it is they want. And it may well be that doctors will have to make some sort of trade-off in spending time in promoting what is in their patients' utility functions and finding out what is there. (This can begin to sound a little incestuous: how much time do patients want their doctors to spend in finding out what patients want?)

Given what has been said about patients not having good information on various aspects of health and health care, it may seem odd to be advocating asking patients what they want. The point is not that they will directly make consumption decisions on this basis. It is that to maximise their utility, or to help them to maximise it, the doctors must know what is relevant to that maximisation. And while the patient may have all sorts of problems in deciding what *weights* to attach to different aspects, it is likely that the patient can form rational judgements about what the arguments are, especially as the health one is obvious and the others may reflect more general aspects of their lives and not be specific to health. Thus an individual's attitude to autonomy is likely to be a general personality trait and not unique to health care decision making. This is likely to be true too of attitudes to information, to dignity, etc.

Of course, patients will, occasionally at least, be directly aware and at other times indirectly aware that there are demands from other patients on their doctor's time. It can be argued that how the doctor decides to deal with this will influence the individual patient's utility. However, I think it is inappropriate for that group of patients, acting as individuals, to try to influence the priority setting in which the doctor has to be involved. This is because the individual patient is too directly involved to be objective about the relative strengths and weaknesses of the different calls on the doctor's time. Further but related, the patients will simply not have the information about other patients to be able to form the necessary judgements.

What this means, importantly, is that at this level it is the doctor – in fact, it *has* to be the doctor – who decides about the opportunity cost of her time. The doctor has to decide whether it is better to spend an extra five minutes with patient A or move on more quickly to patient B. There will, of course, be a lot of uncertainty in making these choices, but it is difficult to see how patients could practically be involved. And in principle it is difficult to see how patients should be involved, i.e. *that* doctor's patients. (There is a case, as will be indicated below, for having patients more generally or society involved in the values that the doctor uses to make these choices and to weigh up the opportunity costs involved. But there seems little justification for trying to bring in that doctor's patients' values in this way.)

There is, however, a rather intriguing aspect to this. Doctors very often argue that they do not want to be involved in consideration of costs. For example, it is possible to pose the question: is it ethical for medical doctors to be involved in consideration of costs? Yet I have just argued that they are, and that they have to be, and that there is no avoiding the issue at least at the level of making choices about the treatment of the patients for whom they are responsible. This may mean that the breadth they attach to the range of forgone opportunities will be rather narrow as compared with some social point of view (an issue I will return to below), but there is no doubt that doctors do consider opportunity cost across their own patients, at least with respect to one key resource (and maybe others) – their own time.

Continually in their decision making doctors have to ask themselves how best to deploy their time and the other resources that are available to them. In doing so they must be weighing up the benefits likely to be obtained from deploying these resources in different ways. And they cannot do that without considering opportunity costs.

Thus, rightly in my view, and ethically (I believe) in their view, doctors are the ones who have to consider costs at this level and indeed they are in my view (and I suspect in theirs as well) the only ones who can do so. This does not mean that they are or ought to be free to use their own values in weighing up the opportunity costs but they are the only ones who are in a position to know what the opportunities are, and practically the only ones who can then exercise the relevant choices. This is certainly true in general practice, although there can be influences clearly from fellow partners and from other practice staff, such as nurses. And it also seems very true in hospital medicine, even if less so, since there is a clearer management structure very often in the hospital sector (although the nature of this is likely to vary from country to country and from health care service to health care service).

What emerges is that doctors are and have to be involved in cost assessment, but where this cost assessment is very clearly based on opportunity cost, i.e. the benefit forgone in using their time elsewhere.

Turning now to the second agency issue – that is, as seen from the standpoint of the wider community – what might perfect agency look like in this context? Here the maximand of agency switches to the social welfare function (i.e. what society wants maximised) rather than the maximisation of patient utility at the more individual level. The issue is rather: what does society want from its health service? The answer would seem to be more complex as it will be looking for an efficient health service – one that maximises the benefit to society of its use of resources – but it will also very likely have some concerns for equity as well. How it is defined is not important, except that it will be concerned with some aspects of distribution as well as maximisation (and there is a need to recognise that the goals of efficiency and equity may at least on occasion conflict). (This issue is dealt with at some length in Chapter 5.)

Precisely how this is handled would seem not to be so much the concern of the medical profession and even less so the concern of the individual doctor. It has to be the case that there cannot be an efficient health service without the involvement of the medical profession since they control or at least influence the use of so many of the resources involved.

When we consider how best to run and organise a health service there may well be the need for an agent at this level in that again the 'citizen' may be poorly informed about how various 'treatments' are likely to work, what the underlying problems are that need to be tackled and what options are available for the 'treatments'. There are parallels between this situation and that which applies at the level of the individual doctor and the treatment of her patients. Clearly we are dealing with wider social issues, but the concept of agency may well apply here as well.

So why cannot the medical doctor operate as the agent for the citizen? There are, I think, three fundamental reasons.

First, the nature of the information gap between the agent and the principal in this case is different. It is about systems and the ways that different forms of health care operate. As such few clinicians are in a position to be any better informed than the majority of the public about these issues (although public health doctors may be).

Second, because this issue lies at this different level, the nature and breadth of 'opportunity cost' is much greater here. Indeed it is unlikely that the doctor will be well placed to form judgements about the opportunity cost at this level. The individual diabetician may well have little idea what the opportunities forgone are as a result of using extra resources to treat diabetes and the obstetrician is likely to be ignorant of the opportunity cost elsewhere in health care as a result of introducing a new prenatal screening test. I would also suggest that there is no reason why clinicians should be interested in these issues. Their responsibility does not lie here.

Third, there is likely to be a clash of interests if clinicians are asked to be agents for their patients and at the same time agents for society. The opportunity costs are different and it is difficult to see how they can be perfect agents at these two levels when the two levels conflict in practice.

This is not to deny the value of agency at this level of the health service. It is simply to state that the role should ideally not be performed by medical doctors who have a continuing responsibility for individual patients. (A more detailed look at what society wants from its health services is deferred to Chapter 11.) Certainly it is an important issue and one that merits much more attention and research than it tends to get or has received in the past.

However, it is relevant here to ponder why there has been this relative neglect. There are two reasons. First, it has perhaps been simply taken for granted that what people want from their health services is only health. Consequently, the idea of trying to find out about people's preferences for what health services might be asked to deliver over and above this has seemed at best superfluous. Second, with the prevailing view – at least among economists – that the key to understanding the nature of health care from an economist's perspective has been the nature of the commodity at the level of the individual purchaser and the individual supplier, the question of health care as a social institution – the nature of this *social* good – has been neglected. Yet with the increasing attention in recent years to 'systems' and the move in many countries to alter the systems (with greater competition, the push on privatisation, etc.) it is perhaps time to get economic researchers and others to look again at the nature of the commodity health care, but this time with at least some greater emphasis on health care as a social institution.

With respect to the perfect agent at this citizen or social level, then the key would seem to lie in getting better information about what citizens want from their health services and then using administrators and policy makers and finally politicians, aided and abetted by public health doctors, to act as the citizens' agents to provide what the society and its citizens want from their health service. It is possible, with the exception of the issue of equity, that what citizens want will essentially be a summation of what patients want. But that at present can only be a guess and the way to remove the guesswork is simply to go out and ask the citizenry: what do you want from your health services?

One other aspect of health care and agency that I would want to touch on here, because it relates to the two levels discussed above (i.e. the individual patient and the individual citizen), is the question of choice. At a time when there is increasing emphasis on the privatisation of health care and increased competition in health care in several countries, there has been a move towards the notion of increased consumer choice. Now I have addressed this issue in greater detail in Chapter 2, dealing with the consumer's utility function. But here I want to consider it very briefly in the wider context of agency. If it is the case that individuals seek greater choice in health care, then I think it is legitimate to allow them to have that greater choice, provided of course that there is a willingness on their part to meet the costs which will be incurred in achieving that greater choice. That is in line with the arguments I have put forward above with respect to the citizens' utility function. If individuals say that they want a health care system to provide them with greater choice, then that is the criterion that would seem appropriate in deciding that that is the way to go.

However, that is not what appears to be happening. There seems to be more of an ideological move to greater choice in health care. This seems to be born of two considerations. First, in recent years there has been a move away from the welfare state of the 1960s and 1970s in a number of countries. There has been a social movement which has seemed to say that welfare is not in a society's interests. Second, there is a simpler ideological view which is not seemingly the same that holds that freedom of choice is a good thing. (There is also a view that greater choice leads to greater efficiency. In Chapter 2 I have tried to point to the problems with that view in the specific context of health care.)

Now there may well be a case for arguing against the featherbedding that the welfare state provided. But I do not see that that argument can automatically be transferred, if at all, into the health care sector. Providing people with health care in a way which gives them greater health is hardly the same type of featherbedding that the opponents of the welfare state would want to criticise. Health or, in this context, illness is different. It may be of course that particular forms of public provision could lead to increased moral hazard, but that does not seem to me to be an argument for choice. It is an argument for reducing moral hazard. (And it should be noted that moral hazard is far from unique to public health care systems and indeed where there is choice – for example, in the United States, with respect to different forms of insurance – there remain large elements of moral hazard. Indeed once insured, moral hazard in the United States is very considerable and I would have difficulties trying to make the case for saying that it is less or greater in the United States than in the more public and socialised systems of Denmark, Sweden or the United Kingdom.) So the argument that choice reduces moral hazard is at best a tortuous one, and one that I do not think can be supported by the evidence that does exist.

With respect to the idea that freedom of choice is a good thing *per se*, it is difficult to argue against this, or at least it is just as difficult to argue for it as it is to argue against it. It is ideological once we remove the possibility that such freedom of choice fosters greater efficiency. It is difficult to 'prove' whether one ideology is better than another. Perhaps again the point would be that the only suitable test of the value of freedom of choice in health care is to ask the citizenry about their preferences for such choice. Presumably those who advocate such a freedom could hardly argue against giving the citizenry the freedom to choose whether they wanted greater freedom of choice in health care or not. There is also, in passing, a very important issue of freedom of choice with respect to what, but that I have left to the discussion in Chapter 11.

Health economists and agency

I have discussed at some length agency and what it might look like when perfect. There has been little written about agency in the context of the citizen, and that is itself interesting and would seem to help to support my call for more research on this topic and more generally consideration of it. It does not seem particularly difficult and, with the sorts of change currently being introduced into health care systems and contemplated, research here would be valuable to help to decide in what directions societies want to head with respect to their health care systems.

Three economists have written about agency at the patient–doctor level at any length, and I want to set out their views here. First, Alan Williams (1988) suggests that a perfect agency relationship would be one where the doctor gave the patient all the information that the patient requires and the patient then makes the decision. The role of the doctor is to overcome the patient's deficiency with respect to information. According to this view the decision remains with the patient. So the patient maximises utility via a process which involves the doctor informing the patient, but that is all the doctor does. Indeed, it is clear from his work elsewhere (Williams, 1985) that he believes that what the patient is trying to maximise is health. In this view, the doctor is providing information to allow the patient to make choices which will maximise health and there are no other arguments in the utility function other than health.

Tony Culyer (1988, 1989) has a somewhat similar view of agency, but rather interestingly takes a different view of who makes the decision. To Culyer it is the doctor who, having informed the patient (again with an apparent restriction to health only as the argument in the utility function), then makes the decision.

In neither Williams' case nor Culyer's is there any allowance for the possibility that information *per se* may be utility or disutility bearing, nor is decision making allowed to be utility or disutility bearing.

Bob Evans (1984) takes a wider view, and argues for the maximand being the utility of the patient. He does not specify what comprises utility for the patient although elsewhere he states that 'Preferences are preferences – economic theory is not supposed to pass moral judgements about what should be in a utility function' (Evans and Wolfson, 1980). My reading of this is that patients can have whatever they want to have as arguments in their utility functions (which clearly coincides with the view expressed in the previous sections about finding out what patients want).

We thus have three leading health economists apparently expressing different views as to what constitutes one of the central concepts of health economics. Such disagreement is worrying, but equally worrying is that there is so little research on the topic. Consequently I would again argue, but still more strongly, for more research on what it is that patients want from their doctors and also what citizens want from their health services.

Before leaving Williams' and Culyer's contributions to agency, a further point to be made is that, as expressed, they seem to leave the potential for agency underexploited. Here is someone (the agent) in a position to try to help the patient in a number of ways and yet they would want to restrict that role to providing information and then about health alone. Their assumptions also mean that the agent is somehow 'invisible' and 'intangible' and indeed makes no mark on the consumption decision or the process involved in that decision, except for the provision of information. That seems both incorrect as a description of practice and simply not possible in practice given the way that medical practitioners do have to interact with their patients. It is difficult, indeed, to see just how this invisible, intangible agent would be able to practise medicine except in theory. What we have here is a very practical tool of health policy which is central to health economics and indeed is central to the practice of medicine in the form of the doctor–patient relationship.

Conclusion

There are all sorts of ways of getting doctors to change their behaviour, and several of these are discussed elsewhere in this book, particularly here and in Chapter 8. Deciding what we want our doctors to do seems to be the challenge of modern health care systems. There is little doubt that if we simply leave doctors to operate as they would wish, then we are unlikely to get the health services that we want. This is not to suggest that doctors are consciously operating contrary to the social interest, but it would only be by chance that behaviour of doctors that was in their best interests would also result in what was best for society. Such things are too important to be left to chance.

To leave such matters to chance would be acceptable, perhaps, if we were dealing with a commodity where there was a balance on the two sides of the market, and suppliers and consumers each had equal power and equal respect for one another. That is not the case in health care and it is worth repeating this again and again to those who advocate competition as the way forward to efficient health care. There may be forms of competition that will work in health care, but any that draw on the philosophy of the private marketplace are almost certainly doomed to fail. Informed choice is the source of the power of the consumer in the private marketplace and informed choice is precisely what the vast majority of patients in the vast majority of circumstances in the market for health care do not have. And it is doubtful even that they want it. It seems more often that patients actively want to rely on an agent whom they hope they can trust. Why try to give them something else based on some ideology of a marketplace which is based on other properties than those that prevail in health care? The economists' belief in the private market is so strong that even when the conditions needed to get markets to work are not there, the blind faith in market forces pushes health care policy makers to close their minds to reason and jump aboard the market bandwagon. The whole basis of the market is that consumers know what they want, know how to get it and through market forces can let suppliers know what they want.

What is needed are incentives so that the trust that patients and citizens want to place in their doctors will be justified and a situation where the doctors, happily maximising their own utilities, also maximise patients' and society's welfare. Getting all three parties to maximise in this way is clearly difficult but it is what we seek. Realising that that is what we seek is the first step.

There is a need to set aside the false gods and inappropriate tools and techniques and get to where the real problems lie. Having identified these, there is then a need to see what the appropriate solutions are. That is the way to get agency as perfect as possible. If we succeed with agency, I think we will be a long way to succeeding with providing the sorts of health services that patients and citizens want.

References

Arrow, K. J. (1986) Agency and the market. In K. J. Arrow and M. D. Intrilligator (eds), *Handbook of Mathematical Economics*, vol. III. Elsevier, Amsterdam.

Culyer, A. J. (1988) Inequality of health services is, in general, desirable. In D. G. Green (ed.), *Acceptable Inequalities*. IEA, London.

Culyer, A. J. (1989) The normative economics of health care financing and provision. *Oxford Review of Economic Policy*, **5**, 34–58.

Evans, R. G. (1984) *Strained Mercy: The economics of Canadian medical care*. Butterworth, Toronto.

Evans, R. G. and Wolfson, A. D. (1980) Faith, hope and charity: health care in the utility function. Discussion paper, Department of Economics, University of British Columbia, Vancouver.

MacDonald, G. M. (1984) New directions in the economic theory of agency. *Canadian Journal of Economics*, **17**, 415–40.

Mooney, G. H. and Ryan, M. (1993) Agency in health care: getting beyond first principles. *Journal of Health Economics*, **12**, 2, 125–35.

Williams, A. (1985) Economics of coronary artery bypass grafting. *British Medical Journal*, **291**, 326–9.

Williams, A. (1988) Priority setting in public and private health care, a guide through the ideological jungle. *Journal of Health Economics*, **7**, 173–83.

7

Does SID exist? And is this the right question?

Introduction

For many years now, and at least since Bob Evans (1974) wrote of the phenomenon twenty years ago, the question of whether 'supplier-induced demand' exists has been a favourite theme of health economists. While there is no consistent definition of SID in the literature, the most common definition would seem to be that of Rice (1983), who defined SID as the extent to which a doctor 'provides or recommends the provision of medical services that differ from what the patient would choose if he or she had available the same information and knowledge as the physician'.

What I want to discuss in this chapter is not whether SID exists or not, but two related questions. First, given Rice's definition, is it possible to prove the existence of SID? And second, is it an important question to address, assuming that it can be answered?

For those readers interested in the controversy as such (i.e. whether or not SID exists), then Feldman and Sloan (1988) and Rice and Labelle (1989) are recommended. Those interested in more detail of the arguments presented here are referred to Ryan and Mooney (1993).

Can SID be tested for?

Examination of the definition of SID reveals that to prove its existence requires showing not only what induced demand looks like but also what *non-induced* demand looks like. According to Rice, the non-induced level of demand corresponds to that which the patient would

104

choose 'if he or she had available the same information and knowledge as the physician'.

The problem that I see here is: at an empirical level how do we establish what this level is? Where would we look for such a level of demand?

One of the major difficulties is that consumers of health care are not as informed or knowledgeable as their doctors. Indeed, this is the very reason why SID, in principle at least, might exist. Yet the definition of SID requires in practice that estimates are made of the level of demand that these informed consumers would have.

One possibility that might be used to circumvent this difficulty is to examine the demand of doctors themselves or doctors' spouses in the belief that (1) they are informed and knowledgeable, and (2) they are presumably less likely to be 'induced' into some level of demand that is different from the one that they as informed patients would choose. However, such patients are not necessarily in other ways typical of what informed patients would like, especially with respect to the sort of value system with which they would operate but also in other ways as well – for example, the social and medical support system with which they operate.

It is perhaps worth recalling at this juncture that the demand for health care is a derived demand resulting largely from the demand for health but such demand need not be restricted to health alone (see Chapter 2). It is therefore based on individuals' valuations of not just health but of other outputs of health care.

It is also relevant to consider that the demand for health care, while a function of the demand for health and these other outputs, is also a function of the perceived effectiveness of health care with respect to these outputs. Thus an individual who perceives the effectiveness of care to be high will *ceteris paribus* demand more health care than one who sees such effectiveness to be low. Individuals may well differ in their demand for health because they value health or health gains differently. They may differ in their demand for health care because they value differently any of the outputs of health care – health, information or whatever. They may have different attitudes to anxiety associated with, say, an operation, or they may differ in their attitudes to risk. They may also be affected by the differing availability or closeness of substitutes for health care such as their family support network or the availability of advice from non-health care sources.

It is clear that the demand for health care is a function of many things. It may well be different even if the individuals concerned have the same health status and have the same set of information with which to make their decision and the same level of knowledge.

It is also to be noted that in empirical studies of SID (see Feldman and Sloan, 1988; Rice and Labelle, 1989) what is used as the variable to estimate demand is not strictly demand but use. Now the relationship between demand and use to be constant across different individuals requires that the costs that the individuals face in using the service are the same. This may well not be the case and indeed it is unlikely that all individuals will have equal access to health care (as is discussed in much greater detail in Chapter 5 on equity). For example, doctors and their spouses are likely to have easier access than the average patient.

There are thus many reasons why we would expect that the demand for health care will vary across different individuals, and even more reasons why we would expect that the use of health services will vary across different individuals even if we standardise for health status and for information and knowledge. What this suggests is that to try to use some proxy for patients whose demand or use we really want to measure rather than the patients themselves would require that we standardise for many other features, including several value-laden features. Consequently, the extent to which we can learn what patients' demand for health care would be if they were as informed and knowledgeable as their doctors by studying the demand of doctors or their spouses, or indeed anyone other than the actual patients when informed, does not seem to be a fruitful way to conduct such analyses.

That leaves the possibility of actually working with informed patients. What is intriguing about the SID literature is that there is no study of which I am aware where patients were informed, their demand (or use) measured in this informed state and this then compared with what actually happened to determine whether what happened differed from what was predicted to happen for these informed patients. In other words, I would suggest that uninduced demand (or use) has never been pinned down empirically. Since that is a prerequisite for any empirical study which sets out to prove whether or not SID exists, I would submit that all existing studies of SID are flawed.

Is this criticism of the whole body of research unjustified? I do not believe so and have argued this position in greater depth (Ryan and Mooney, 1993). Indeed, the literature on SID at an empirical level is singularly silent on the question of what non-induced demand looks like.

That raises the interesting question of why such an odd circumstance can arise. The answer – which was also encountered in Chapter 5 on equity – is that there is again a tendency here to 'move the target to hit the bullet' in the words of Bob Evans, writing from another context. In other words, because it is too difficult to measure what we want to measure, economists measure something else (a phenomenon that also exists in the context of equity – see Chapter 5). As uninduced demand cannot easily, if at all, be measured and to date at least has not been measured, then let us measure something else.

Of course, in research such a tactic is wholly legitimate provided that there is a recognition of what is being done and that there is some thought given to whether the proxy is a reasonable approximation to whatever it is that is being investigated. However, there is little recognition of this problem in the literature on SID and that would seem to be a rather important criticism not only of SID *per se* and whether it exists or not, but also of the researchers who have worked on this issue.

Whither SID?

The question then arises: what should be done with respect to future research on SID and its possible existence? Can the problems indicated in the last section be overcome, and if so how? And more fundamentally perhaps, whether they can or not, is it worth trying to overcome these problems, or is there some other related research agenda which it might be better to pursue?

On the first issue I cannot see that the problems can be overcome without a truly enormous and very detailed study requiring that potential patients be informed to the same level as their doctors (and establishing what that level might be would in itself be difficult). The same would be required with respect to knowledge and that seems even more difficult. (While the distinction between information and knowledge is not always clear, I think it is useful to consider that while information can be conveyed, it only becomes knowledge if it is understood and retained by the recipient for future possible use. There is an important distinction between the two and trying to alter levels of knowledge is likely to prove more difficult than altering information levels; assessing levels of knowledge is also likely to prove more difficult than with information.)

However, assuming that the patients could be informed and made knowledgeable to the required extent, it would be possible to determine what their level of use was. Provided that we could be sure that their access to care was the same, we would be able to assess whether their use differed according to whether it was 'uninduced' or 'induced', with the former being their use without contact with the doctor and the latter being their use with contact with the doctor. But how would we get a level of use which did not involve contact with the doctor?

There seems no way out of the problem even if we were prepared to undertake very large and expensive studies to determine whether SID exists or not. It just seems impossible to measure uninduced demand satisfactorily. Consequently, if uninduced demand cannot be measured satisfactorily, it is difficult to see how the existence of SID can be measured in practical terms.

Does it matter that we cannot apparently test for the presence of SID in practice? Fortunately I think it does not, and indeed in terms of the relations between economists and doctors, perhaps if economists stopped trying to prove that doctors indulge in inducement the relations between the two disciplines might improve! There has been a moralistic tone to at least some of the research on SID and suggestions that inducement is unethical in some sense or other. One benefit of stopping further research on SID would be that this form of challenging of the ethics of the profession would cease.

More importantly it would mean that economists could concentrate on what is likely to prove to be the more important issue, viz. if doctors are not doing what society wants them to do, how do we provide incentives to get them to change their practices? Whether this involves inducement ceases to be the issue. All we require is to determine how practical it is to get doctors to change their practices and how this change can be brought about most efficiently.

As discussed in Chapter 8 on medical practice variations, the issues are how to get doctors to practise efficiently and also how to define efficiency in this context. What this means in essence is getting agreement with the profession that efficiency matters and in turn that best medical practice is to be equated with efficient medical practice.

That may or may not seem obvious. Certainly I cannot see how we can get efficient health services without having efficient doctors. And there is good evidence that doctors are prepared to alter their practice as a result of facing different patterns of incentives. The point is to get agreement on what they are to do in society's wider interests and put the appropriate set of incentives in place to get them to act efficiently in pursuit of these social objectives.

Such comments might be interpreted in some quarters – and especially by medical doctors – as an attack on doctors' current inefficiency. It is not intended as such. I am clear that it is most unlikely that doctors, left to their own devices, will practise efficiently. This is not intentional in the sense that they deliberately set out to be inefficient. But very often doctors do not understand what efficiency means in an economic sense, or perhaps worse have experienced situations which make them believe that efficiency is to be equated with cost cutting. Certainly, doctors are often suspicious of the concept of efficiency and to some extent with some justification, given the way that many health services, and health service management in particular, have misused the concept of efficiency to mean economising. Once the notion of efficiency is accepted by the profession in its true economic sense – the eventual maximisation of benefit from the resources available – then it is likely that doctors will be more willing to embrace efficiency.

Efficiency at the clinical level will, however, be primarily in the form of operational efficiency – attempting to meet particular objectives, at least cost – although there will inevitably be some aspects of allocative efficiency present as well, i.e. clinicians will have to judge which objectives to meet and to what extent and at the expense of which others. But it is operational efficiency that will tend to dominate.

The position is not helped by the fact that there is normally very poor or non-existent data on costs at the clinical level. Some (such as those generated by DRGs – see Chapter 10) are likely to be positively misleading and if used by clinicians, may result in their being led away from efficiency rather than closer to it.

It is also the case that on the benefit or output side there has been too little effort from the profession to try to grapple with the measurement of health so that even today we still see many studies of clinical effectiveness which measure output in very crude terms such as mortality only, or survival over, say, five years. Again, there are signs of change but it is a most peculiar facet of medical practice not only with respect to efficiency but with respect to effectiveness that the profession has been so slow to show any great interest in measurement of what it is that they are trying to produce.

We know too little about efficiency at the clinical level largely because there have been relatively few studies conducted to assess the efficiency of clinical procedures through the use, for example, of cost-effectiveness and cost-utility analyses. Gerard (1992), in her review of cost-utility studies in the English language in the period from 1980 to mid-1991, could find only fifty-one published studies. Given the way in which she tackled this it is unlikely that many were missed. Many more such studies are needed if there is to be improvement in the efficiency of clinical procedures.

Why is so little currently being done? First, there have been too few clinicians interested in efficiency, largely because there is little concern and even less incentive to be interested in clinical efficiency. Why under most health care systems should clinicians be anxious or even care about their use of resources? Neither they nor their patients are likely to benefit through straining to be efficient. Second, the nature of the funding arrangements in most health care systems does not encourage doctors to think about the way in which they use the resources at their disposal. Third, it is often difficult for the doctors to gain any insight into what resources they do use, and that is no great encouragement to them to improve efficiency. Fourth, the emphasis in clinical medicine is largely on effectiveness and most clinical trials only get that far, and resource use is not included in the data collected in evaluations from such trials. There are signs of change on this front but they are slow. (For example, in the United Kingdom at least there are a few tentative and very shaky steps being taken by the Medical Research Council to try to get health economists more involved in economic evaluations of clinical trials. Unfortunately, they have thought too little about how to get the successful involvement of these health economists and seemingly not at all about how the medical fraternity might be expected to react to such 'interference' in 'their' evaluations from this outside and largely unwelcome discipline.) Fifth, the move to improve medical practice through audit is concerned almost exclusively with effectiveness, and indeed it is sometimes argued by medical auditors that efficiency is not their concern; that is for someone else to deal with. (That may well be a valid point but there do seem dangers in leaving the definition of best medical practice wholly to non-doctors and that is what might happen if doctors refuse to accept some responsibility for defining efficiency in clinical prac- tice.)

There would thus seem to be a strong case for mounting many more studies to investigate clinical efficiency. This would seem a better use of economists' time than the pursuit of truth surrounding the existence or non-existence of SID. But additionally there is a need to investigate more thoroughly what the impact of different forms of incentives are on doctors' behaviour. Certainly, there is good evidence to show that doctors do behave differently when the incentive structure they face changes. But we know too little about the impact of such incentives.

As is indicated in Chapter 9 on patient payment and paying doctors there are ways of getting doctors to change, and it is with the behaviour of doctors rather than of patients that we must place our faith when trying to devise policy for promoting efficiency in health care. There is no symmetry in health care with respect to the supply side and the demand side. Doctors do have a greater influence on what patients demand than do suppliers in other markets. But the message here is that we must pin our hopes on the doctors for the promotion of efficiency in health care. It is they who can help patients to adopt more efficient roles; indeed they have a responsibility to do so.

But in the end the key to this issue of promoting efficiency through altering doctor behaviour rests on devising incentives which will result in doctors maximising their utility at the same time as they promote social efficiency. That is the key goal of health policy. Yet it is one that economists working in health care have paid too little attention to. They have tended to dismiss fee-for-service (FFS) medicine as resulting in 'over-servicing', and neglected the fact that whatever incentives are present in FFS medicine will undoubtedly be affected by the level of the fees and not just the existence of fees. They have also seemingly neglected the substantial body of literature in mainstream economics which deals with agency. That literature points to the fact that to achieve anything equating to even an approximation of perfect agency requires very complex fee arrangements. If that is true outside medicine, then it is likely to be even more true in health care. What is needed is a major research programme from economists with their clinical colleagues to address the best way of paying our doctors – but only after there has been a debate among policy makers and perhaps the community more generally as to what the objectives of health care are to be.

Conclusion

Some of the aspects discussed in this chapter are taken up in more detail and from different perspectives in Chapter 9 on paying doctors and paying patients and in Chapter 11 on what we can expect from our doctors. What I have concentrated on here is demonstrating that the question of whether or not SID exists is not important. In so far as it is clear that doctors can influence what patients do and what services they take up and therefore what resources they consume, then it becomes important to establish what society wants the doctors to do. So the first task is to determine what is efficient medical practice. Thereafter there is a need for more research to establish how different forms of incentives influence doctors and then move to implement a structure of incentives which will get doctors doing what is efficient for their patients and beyond that for society more generally.

This is the task and not the pursuit of trying to pin down whether or not SID exists – even if it were possible to do that, which I would submit it is not.

References

Evans, R. G. (1974) Supplier-induced demand: some empirical evidence and implications. In M. Perlman (ed.), *The Economics of Health and Medical Care*. North-Holland, Amsterdam.

Feldman, R. and Sloan, F. (1988) Competition among physicians, revisited. *Journal of Health Politics, Policy and Law*, **13**, 2, 239–61.

Gerard, K. (1992) Cost-utility in practice: a policy maker's guide to the state of the art. *Health Policy*, **21**, 3, 1–31.

Rice, T. H. (1983) The impact of changing medicare reimbursement rates on physician-induced demand. *Medical Care*, **21**, 8, 803–15.

Rice, T. H. and Labelle, R. J. (1989) Do physicians induce demand for medical services? *Journal of Health Politics, Policy and Law*, **14**, 3, 587–600.

Ryan, M. and Mooney, G. H. (1993) Supplier induced demand: an agenda for future research. Mimeo, Health Economics Research Unit, University of Aberdeen, Aberdeen.

8

Medical practice variations

Introduction

One of the most fascinating and almost certainly inefficient and inequitable aspects of modern medicine is the extent and nature of variation in medical practice. It is a blight on the medical landscape. Yet the extent to which policy has moved to deal with variations is surprisingly small.

There are substantial variations in the way that doctors treat what appear to be the same illnesses. While one would expect some variation, reflecting, for example, differences among patients in their wishes and preferences, the fact that much of the existing variation seems to be a function of the doctor rather than the patient has to be a cause for concern. It is the evidence at the level of populations – 'market areas' such as hospital catchment areas as they have been called (Wennberg and Gittelsohn, 1973) – that gives rise to most concern. The main explanation for these variations lies in differences in the way that doctors are treating what are ostensibly similar populations of patients.

The extent to which this may be seen as problematical is still greater when it is appreciated that patients will be little aware (if at all) of such variations. Further, patients are unlikely – even if they had general knowledge of the existence of variations – to be able to tell where their doctor is on any spectrum of variations for the treatment of the condition they have. In fact, it is unlikely that in other than a few instances the doctor will be able to place him or herself on that spectrum! Even today, when talking to doctors about such variations, some will try strenuously to deny their existence or attempt to come up with explanations which would be less threatening to the medical profession. Indeed, one of the most interesting aspects of this issue of variations is the extent to which doctors seem to find admitting to their existence a threat.

In this chapter I want to look at the extent and nature of such variations and consider what if anything might or should be done about them. I will consider these aspects principally from the perspective of efficiency, but also touch on equity aspects as well. In the next section I set out the evidence on variations and discuss the conflicting theories that exist with respect to why these variations exist. I will then turn to considerations of the policy implications of variations, particularly addressing the question of what policy makers might do about them. This will bring me into the realm of medical audit since it is here that I feel that the profession may be failing to realise the full potential that exists both for variations to create major problems for them and their patients and for the profession to act to reduce variations and thereby promote both efficiency and equity in health care.

Variations: background and evidence

Knowledge of the existence of variations in medical practice has been with us for at least fifty years (Glover, 1938) but it is in the last twenty-five years that research has revealed that almost no matter what procedure one looks at and in which country there is substantial variation in the way that doctors practise. For some of the best early studies see, for example, Pearson *et al.* (1968) and Bunker (1970).

McPherson (1990) has suggested that there are five possible sources of variations in medical procedures across different populations. These are morbidity; those that are random; availability and supply; clinical; and demand. While each of these can contribute to variations in medical practice across different populations, some may be seen or interpreted as more 'legitimate' than others. For example, if morbidity varies, then of course we would expect there to be variations in rates of interventions to deal with such morbidity. However, where the explanation lies in variations between doctors in the way that they treat similar patients (and such variations are not known to the patients concerned), then this is a less legitimate form of variation, particularly in health care systems that seek to pursue objectives of efficiency and equity. This is expressed particularly well by Mulley (1990) and I shall quote him at length:

> Practice variation, *measured from case to case*, may reflect differences in valuations made by different people (or *for* different people) for the same

health outcomes. When the purpose of the intervention is to improve the quality of life, preferences and underlying values may be the critical variables in determining whether the procedure is indicated or not. Such variability is desirable and should be preserved. For most variable procedures and interventions, it is unlikely that the populations' distributions of preferences for relevant outcomes are sufficiently different to explain observed variation. More likely, providers in areas with different rates have different preferences and/or attitudes towards risk, and their views (overly) influence the decision; the agency role is inadequate for the complex communication tasks necessary to allow adequate definition of patient preferences so that the choice made will be consistent with the relevant utility and attitudes towards risk. (emphasis in original)

In other words, differences in doctors' values will be reflected in differences in medical practice.

Mulley seems to sum up the different sources of variation neatly. However, I think that part of the explanation for variations may be that what doctors are trying to do to patients may differ, i.e. their objectives are different or as a minimum the weights they attach to the different possible objectives they have differ. Now it may be that Mulley intended that this aspect of possible sources of variation should be encompassed within his comment that doctors have 'different preferences' but the issue of different objectives seems to go a stage further. So it would follow that the importance Mulley places on the agency role while not misplaced might be missing out on the fact that the interpretation of the agency role by different doctors might be quite different. This might be in terms of what it is that the doctor is trying to maximise on behalf of the patient – for example, is it health or some wider concept of utility or patient satisfaction? (See Chapter 6 for more discussion of the agency role in health care.) Thus aspects of patient care, such as respect for patient autonomy and the provision of information, are not simply matters of preference with respect to quality of life but raise important issues regarding what the objectives of medical practice are.

Despite the evidence, there seems too little recognition in policy making in health care of these variations and too little recognition of the possible policy benefits – health benefits in the end – to be obtained by getting to grips with variations. For example, Evans (1990) writes:

Knowing is not the same as doing. The most striking fact about the large and extensively documented variations in patterns of medical practice, throughout the developed world, is the minimal impact this information has had on health policy.

There are variations across countries and within countries. At the former level, for example, Pearson *et al.* (1968) found that rates of admission to hospital were consistently higher in the United States than in the United Kingdom. However, when Sweden was considered, that country's rates showed less consistency *vis-à-vis* the United Kingdom and the United States, with some rates being similar to those in the United States and others sometimes even lower than in the United Kingdom. Even within Scandinavia Hoyer (1985) found very substantial variations in rates of compulsory admission to psychiatric hospitals in 1982: Sweden 248 per 100,000 population, Norway 109 and Denmark 26. (This may well be more a reflection of socio-cultural values than strictly medical values in these countries.)

Within countries there are at least as substantial variations. There is a sixfold variation in hysterectomy rates for benign indications in Denmark across hospital catchment areas (Andersen *et al.*, 1987) and a 3-5-fold variation in tonsillectomy rates within countries (McPherson *et al.*, 1982). Of a US study Wennberg *et al.* (1987) write:

> Residents of New Haven are about twice as likely to undergo a bypass operation for coronary artery disease as their counterparts in Boston, who are more likely to be treated by other means. On the other hand, Bostonians are much more likely to have their hips and knees replaced by a surgical prosthesis than are New Havenites, whose physicians tend to prescribe medical treatment for these conditions. Bostonians are twice as likely to have a carotid endarterectomy . . .

And so on and so on.

It seems that for every country and every procedure investigated these sorts of variations in medical practice exist.

Certainly, the extent of variation varies from country to country and from procedure to procedure (with those where there is less scope for discretion, such as appendectomy, varying less). There is some limited evidence (see McPherson *et al.*, 1982) to suggest that FFS medicine may result in greater variations than under systems with other forms of doctor remuneration. The evidence, however, is scant and, as is implied in Chapter 9 on paying doctors, much will depend on the nature of the fee schedule rather than on the existence of FFS *per se*.

Theories

Despite the weight of evidence for the existence of variations accumulated over more than half a century, the extent to which variations have been subject to investigatory studies to try to explain their existence is rather limited. Certainly there has been a plethora of studies showing the existence of variations. There is less – much less – on the explanatory front. Here I want to examine two competing theories and offer some observations on their rival merits. Which theory is more accurate seems to matter. Each points to different policy prescriptions, and there is thus a need to choose which theory to run with if the issues of variations at a policy level are to be addressed.

Wennberg (1984) has advanced the theory that the explanation for medical practice variations rests with what he calls 'the professional uncertainty hypothesis'. This is summed up by Mulley (1990):

> This hypothesis holds that when geographical variation cannot be explained by disease prevalence, access to and availability of services, or enabling factors such as insurance, it reflects differences in physicians' beliefs about the value of the variable procedures and practices for meeting patients' needs. The uncertainty may result from inadequate information on the part of some professionals when the information is known to others, or may reflect the real limits of medical knowledge at the time.

Evans (1990), on the other hand, puts forward what might be described as the professional disagreement hypothesis. This is in essence the view that doctors are not necessarily uncertain about what they are doing; it is more that they disagree about what is best.

Now following this through in more detail (see Mooney and Ryan, 1993), three features are relevant. First, doctors may have different objectives in mind when treating their patients. Second, they may have the same objectives but in making choices about treatments they may disagree about which method is best to achieve the objective because they operate on the basis of different information. Third, they may disagree about which method is best to achieve the objective because, while operating on the basis of the same information, the values they use to interpret the information are different.

Evidence on whether doctors are attempting to achieve different things when treating their patients is rather thin. This seems not to have been a question that researchers have been very interested to answer. It may be, of course, that there has been an assumption that such a question simply was not worthy of investigation. After all, why would doctors have different objectives? Are they not all trying to do the best for their patients?

There is evidence that doctors can change their minds about what they have been doing as a result of having it pointed out to them what some of the implications are of their actions. For example, in Finland the evidence from a study by Holli and Hakama (1989, 1990) on changes over time in the treatment of breast cancer patients seems to suggest that doctors moved from being concerned almost solely with treating the disease to a broader concern with patient welfare. But there seems to be less information in the literature more generally on the variations across doctors in what they are trying to do.

As indicated in Chapter 6 on agency, there is a need to investigate more generally what doctors' objectives are and what they interpret the arguments in the patients' utility functions to be. In particular I am thinking here of the extent to which patients have arguments beyond health in their utility functions and whether doctors attempt to find out about these arguments.

The second issue noted above – that doctors have the same objectives but have different information available in choosing which treatment to recommend – is closest to the Wennberg uncertainty hypothesis. However, it is worthy of note that while Wennberg concentrates on the uncertainty surrounding effectiveness of care, i.e. what the impact of treatment is on the health status of the patient, as set out here there is scope for allowing uncertainty to range across a wider set of variables. Thus possible areas where there could be different information sets available to doctors would include the following:

1. The range of treatments from which to choose. There may be some treatments which some doctors simply do not know about or which they fail to consider because of 'biases' against them, e.g. the possibility of addiction with, say, sleeping pills.
2. The cost of treatments (and the extent to which cost affects the doctor's decision – either because of different resource constraints or because of different perceptions of the relevance of cost to clinical decision making).
3. Other aspects of the treatment not included in 1 or 2 above, which perhaps can best be placed under the heading of 'process variables'. These might include such factors as inconvenience to patients; possible side effects; and painfulness or other negative aspects of care. In other words, these might be considered as aspects of effectiveness when effectiveness is defined more broadly than just the impact on the health status with respect to the problem as diagnosed.

Now as indicated, the Wennberg 'professional uncertainty' hypothesis can be incorporated into the second 'disagreement' hypothesis. But there is much more to the second theory than to the first.

Does it matter which we choose? The answer, I think, depends on why we want to know in the first place. I would suggest that the key reason for trying to understand medical practice variations is to consider whether, first, they are in some sense 'important', and second, they run counter to some or other objective in health care. Thereafter, if that is the case, then there is a need to consider how best policy instruments can be devised to reduce the extent of variations in some efficient way.

There seems little doubt that medical practice variations are important and in a negative way. For example, Wennberg has indicated, again for the study of New Haven and Boston quoted earlier (Wennberg *et al.*, 1987) that:

> Bostonians are much more likely to be hospitalised for medical conditions than are their counterparts who live in New Haven. In 1982 Medicare reimbursements for hospitals were $1894 in Boston per person, while in New Haven they were $1078. If New Haven reimbursements had applied to the 78,000 enrollees living in Boston, the outlays would have been $63 million less – $85 million rather than the actual $148 million.

This is simply one assessment of their importance in cost terms. Since we do not know what the optimal level of activity is, it would be wrong to think that this is necessarily the best way to represent the size of the problem. It might be better – but the information is not available – to present information about the health shortfall as a result of 'underprovision' of services or procedures. We cannot do that, however.

What seems clear is that not all doctors can be practising efficient care. Indeed, the majority are likely to be practising inefficient care to a greater or lesser extent – even if we do not know which doctors these are since we do not know what efficient care levels are.

So medical practice variations are a source of inefficiency in health care. It is probably the case that they are a major source of inefficiency, but that is more difficult to prove.

But given the nature of the variations it is likely that they lead to substantial inequities in health care. This is most readily seen if it is the case that we are content to measure inequities in terms of variations in utilisation rates. In so far as variations exist which are to do solely with the supply-side variation in doctors, then variations in medical practice are themselves directly indicators of the extent of inequities across different areas.

We thus have the information available to show that variations in medical practice run counter to the two main objectives of health care – efficiency and equity. We thus have established the key argument for the study of variations and why we need to understand them.

With respect to policy instruments to deal with variations, which theory is correct or which theory 'fits better' will provide pointers to policy in dealing with variations. In other words, the theory underlying and explaining variations should help in the process of selecting the appropriate policy instruments.

Wennberg's emphasis in policy terms, given his concern with the professional uncertainty surrounding effectiveness, is not surprisingly to concentrate on getting more information about effectiveness and making sure that doctors have that information. The assumption here seems to be that if the doctors have that information, they will adjust their behaviour accordingly and the extent of variation will decline. Wennberg assumes that all doctors want to practise good medicine and that, but for their ignorance of the effectiveness of their care, they would agree as to what that good practice is.

Evans, on the other hand, argues that doctors are certain – each is certain – that what he or she is doing is right. The fact that his or her colleagues are doing something else is not an issue, far less a problem. Clinical freedom allows individual doctors to decide what is best for their patients. The fact that Dr Paul is doing something different from Dr Peter is deemed not relevant to Dr Paul or Dr Peter, or any other doctor for that matter. (We are not talking about ethics here, and the variations are assumed to be within what would be deemed ethical limits at the present time.)

When it comes to policy prescriptions there is some limited evidence that Wennberg's view does not work – that as professional uncertainty is the root cause of medical practice variations it is information with respect in particular to effectiveness that is needed to get doctors to change their behaviour. This policy is embodied in the view that the way to get clinicians to come into line with good practice and to reduce variations in clinical practice is to promulgate standards of care, and it is this that has prompted so much of the work on medical audit, model health care programmes, clinical guidelines, reference programmes, etc. in various countries in recent years. There is little evidence that such guidelines and standards are effective in changing clinicians' behaviour. For example, Lomas (1990) argues that 'it will not be long before it becomes widely known that standards set from afar, and labelled only as guidelines, are changing little out in the field of medical practice'.

In arguing against the professional uncertainty hypothesis, Evans suggests that if uncertainty were the answer, then clinicians would warmly embrace any new information that would help to reduce their uncertainty. He claims, however, that they do not: 'The surgeons who scrawl their surgical signatures across Wennberg's data sets, the hospital prone physicians identified by Roos *et al.* (1986) who maintain the hospital industry of Manitoba, are not at all uncertain about the rightness of what they are doing.'

It may simply be, however, that inadequate efforts have been made to get the evidence rather than that the Evans hypothesis is to be deemed the more accurate. What matters beyond this is what the two different policy prescriptions would be and what, if they worked, they would be likely to achieve. So let us switch to the issue of what we want any policy related to variations to achieve.

The argument against practice variations so far has been that they are inefficient and inequitable. How do policy makers improve the promotion of the goals of efficiency and equity through dealing with variations? What, if doctors are doing different things, do we want doctors to do?

The answer to the latter question seems to be 'to practise best medicine' where best medicine is defined in terms of efficiency and equity. Let us leave the equity issue to one side for the moment and concentrate on efficiency.

One major drawback in defining best medical practice in terms of efficiency is that for the great majority of medical practice we do not have information about its effectiveness, never mind its efficiency. But that does not mean that we should not try to define best medical practice in these terms.

What is needed is a wide range of studies to determine what is efficient practice. This seems so obvious yet there is little support, apparently, for such a move (although in the pharmaceutical field starts are being made in going down this road, especially in Australia).

In other words there is a need to decide what we want doctors to do – and not just think about narrowing the variations in what they do do. After all, such narrowing could conceivably result in greater inefficiencies depending on where efficient practice lies in the range.

Beyond identifying where we want doctors to be, the challenge shifts to getting doctors there in the most cost-effective way.

Information seems insufficient. Consequently, we need to examine incentives for getting doctors to change their behaviour, and there is evidence that doctors do change their behaviour as a result of changes in their remuneration system. There may well be incentives other than financial reward to doctors, but the evidence is less clear-cut.

On financial incentives there would seem to be clear arguments for operating a system of at least part-FFS medicine. Many economists seem to think that FFS medicine will inevitably lead to 'overtreatment', although since it is frequently difficult to define optimal treatment, it is difficult to know and to diagnose overtreatment. But more fundamentally still, there is no reason *per se* to think that FFS will automatically get doctors to do more than they would under other remuneration systems. Much depends on the fee schedule.

Elsewhere (see Chapter 9) I have discussed doctor remuneration. The key issues, however, would seem to be these: there is evidence to show that doctors behave differently under different remuneration systems. We know that changing their remuneration systems alters, or can alter, their behaviour. However, our knowledge of which remuneration changes have which effects is more limited. More experimentation with doctor remuneration is needed and more acceptance among policy makers of just how powerful a tool doctor remuneration can and should be.

Doctors are likely to perform more of certain procedures if they are paid higher fees per minute (net, after allowing for the costs that doctors face in conducting the procedures). Paying doctors FFS for some items and not others, or varying the return per minute, can affect the distribution of doctors' time over different procedures and conceivably also the distribution of the activities *per se*.

There is a need for much greater research into the effects of different remuneration systems but also into variations within systems, especially with respect to the fee schedule of FFS systems. What has an effect on what doctors do and how they spend their time is almost certainly complex. The crude 'FFS means overservicing' reaction of health economists is far too simplistic.

Perhaps still more fundamentally there is a need for greater recognition – and indeed acceptance – in the profession, but even more so among the policy makers and the general public, that the idea of giving doctors incentives to act in ways that are in the interests of society and which they might not otherwise do is not a problem in any sort of ethical terms. It may well be that we would like our doctors to transcend such things as concerns for their incomes. But why should they? Why in this respect should they be different from the rest of us? There is every reason to allow doctors to try to maximise their utility, although at the same time trying to get them to maximise their patients' utility and the social welfare. It is difficult to try to pursue these three goals at one and the same time, and may be impossible to meet them all. It is inevitable that the doctor will be more concerned about the patients she sees and her family and herself. So the task of health policy makers is not to become frustrated or annoyed that doctors want to do that, but rather to use these motivations in a positive way. There are bound to be conflicts of interests and concerns, so rather than bemoan that, the point in policy terms would be to try to use these conflicting motivations positively.

Readers may interpret this as meaning that doctors can legitimately act in their own selfish interests and only be conscious of the wishes of their patients when it suits them financially or in other ways that increase their utility. That is not my point; but in so far as that does happen, I think it should be used positively. I would still want the members of the medical profession to be trained in a way that results in their emerging as caring people who are interested in the health and welfare of their patients. I would still want it to be the case that there is an interdependence in the utility functions of doctors and patients in the sense that when patients do well, doctors get utility from that and when things go wrong for patients doctors feel badly about it. While much of this may well be cultural in the sense of being part of the social values in any society, I think that at least some aspects of these caring values can be helped and encouraged, especially in the process of the early training of doctors and perhaps also in the selection of entrants for medical school.

References

Andersen, T. F., Madsen, M. and Loft, A. (1987) Regionale variationer i anvendelsen af hysterektomi (Regional variations in hysterectomy rates). *Ugeskrift for Lager*, **36**, 149, 2415–9.

Bunker, P. (1970) Surgical manpower. A comparison of operations and surgeons in the United States and in England and Wales. *New England Journal of Medicine*, **282**, 3, 941–73.

Evans, R. G. (1990) The dog in the night-time: medical practice variations and health policy. In T. F. Andersen and G. Mooney (eds) *The Challenges of Medical Practice Variations*. Macmillan, London.

Glover, J. A. (1938) The incidence of tonsillectomy in school children. *Proceedings of the Royal Society of Medicine*, **31**, 1219–36.

Holli, K. and Hakama, M. (1989) Treatment of the terminal stages of breast cancer. *British Medical Journal*, **298**, 13–14.

Holli, K., Hakama, M. and Mooney, G. (1990) Changing clinical practice: a case study in breast cancer. In U. J. Jensen and G. Mooney (eds) *Changing Values in Medical and Health Care Decision Making*. Wiley, London.

Hoyer, G. (1985) Tvangsinnleggelser og tvangsretensjon i psykiatriske institusjoner – en sammenligning av regelverk og praksis i de skandinaviske land (Compulsory admissions to psychiatric institutions – a comparison of regulations and practice across Scandinavian countries). *Nordisk Psykiatrisk Tidsskrift*, **39**, 147–57.

Lomas, J. (1990) Promoting clinical policy change: using the art to promote the science in medicine. In T. F. Andersen and G. Mooney (eds), *The Challenges of Medical Practice Variations*. Macmillan, London.

McPherson, K. (1990) Why do variations occur? In T. F. Andersen and G. Mooney (eds), *The Challenges of Medical Practice Variations*. Macmillan, London.

McPherson, K., Wennberg, J. E., Hovind, O. and Clifford, P. (1982) Small area variations in the use of common surgical procedures: an international comparison of New England, England and Norway. *New England Journal of Medicine*, **307**, 1310–14.

Mooney, G. and Ryan, M. (1993) Agency in health care; getting beyond first principles. *Journal of Health Economics*, **12**, 2, 125–35.

Mulley, A. G. (1990) Medical decision making and practice variation. In T. F. Andersen and G. Mooney (eds), *The Challenges of Medical Practice Variations*. Macmillan, London.

Pearson, R. J. C., Smedby, B., Bertenstam, R., Logan, R. F., Burgess, A. M. and Peterson, O. L. (1968) Hospital caseloads in Liverpool, New England and Uppsala. An international comparison. *The Lancet*, 7 September, 559–66.

Roos, N. P., Flowerdew, G., Wajda, A. and Tate, R. B. (1986) Variations in physicians' hospitalization practices: a population based study in Manitoba, Canada. *American Journal of Public Health*, **76**(1), 45–51.

Wennberg, J. E. (1984) Dealing with medical practice variations: a proposal for action. *Health Affairs*, **3**, 2, 6–32.

Wennberg, J. E. and Gittelsohn, A. (1973) Small area variations in health care delivery: a population-based health information system can guide planning and regulatory decision making. *Science*, **182**, 1102–9.

Wennberg, J. E., Freeman, J. L. and Culp, W. J. (1987) Are hospital services rationed in New Haven or over-utilized in Boston? *The Lancet*, 23 May, 1185–9.

9

Paying doctors – and non-paying patients

Introduction

Two key issues in health policy are: how to pay doctors and whether patients should pay at the point of consumption (and if so how). In this chapter I have taken the two issues together because I think they are about providing incentives to the two key sets of actors on the health care stage and as such merit being considered together. This is not done sufficiently often in my view and there are clear advantages in doing so.

In the next section I will indicate what I see as some of the more important issues in doctor remuneration and include there some results of research in which I have been directly involved and which has persuaded me that fee-for-service (FFS) medicine is not, or at least not always, the curse that many economists seem to assume. If it does, as is sometimes claimed, lead to over-servicing, then if we are to form a reasoned judgement of that we need to know what 'optimal servicing' is. That seems not to be known. Thus while it may well be that certain forms of FFS medicine will lead to excess supply, other forms can inject social priorities into medical decision making which might be rather different from the priorities that the profession would otherwise pursue.

Thereafter I want to look at the implications of patient payments for both efficiency and equity in health care. There are better – and worse – ways of getting patients to pay depending on what it is that health policy makers seek to achieve. Perhaps the best way is not to have them pay at all or to offer financial inducements – negative patient payments – in certain instances to increase the use of health services or to improve access to health services. This issue will be debated in the third section of this chapter.

Finally, I want to bring these two issues together and think through how best they can be combined to get efficient and/or equitable health care. We have here the two key actors – the doctor and the patient. What combination of incentives can best provide what it is that health services are trying to achieve?

Paying doctors

In a study in Denmark in which I was involved (Krasnik *et al.*, 1990), we were able to examine the way in which a change in the remuneration system affected the way that doctors – in this case GPs – practice medicine. There were two rather remarkable things about the study. First, it was conducted against a background of considerable ignorance of how such changes in doctor remuneration affect how they act – an ignorance which, although a little less common now, remains remarkably widespread, given how important the issue is in health policy terms. Second, while the direction of the changes in behaviour that did occur was somewhat predictable, what was certainly not predicted was the magnitude of the changes. (I report in detail on the study below.) Doctors are influenced by how they are paid. Just how big that influence is is the key message that emerges from the study.

Prior to October 1987, general practitioners (GPs) in Copenhagen City were paid very largely on a capitation basis, unlike their counterparts in the rest of Denmark, who were paid partly on a capitation basis and partly by FFS. After October 1987 the Copenhagen City GPs moved to the same remuneration system as the rest of the country's GPs.

Under the FFS system GPs were paid fees for face-to-face consultations, telephone consultations, repeat prescriptions and home visits. They received additional fees for performing certain services to patients, such as cervical smears, removal of wax from ears, blood tests, etc.

The study to examine the effects of the change on the behaviour of the Copenhagen City GPs was based on the results of a special survey of seventy-one randomly selected GPs in Copenhagen City for one period before the change (March 1987) and two periods after the change (March 1988 and November 1988). Each period covered all patient contacts in a particular week. These results were compared with the activities of GPs in Copenhagen County (the control group). Two periods were used after the change because it was thought that

Table 9.1   Number of contacts and activities in a week and number of enlisted patients in March 1987, March 1988 and November 1988 for seventy-one doctors in Copenhagen City.

	March 1987	March 1988	November 1988
Contacts	9,942	11,387	10,618
Diagnostic services*	536	768	896
Curative services*	99	201	203
Referrals to specialist	1,276	1,176	1,002
Referrals to hospital	251	226	176
Number of enlisted patients	122,223	125,412	125,536

*Services for which additional fee is paid.

the change might not be the same in the immediate aftermath of the switch in remuneration systems as in a later period when the GPs would have had more time to adjust to the effects of the remuneration change.

Tables 9.1, 9.2 and 9.3 report on the changes that occurred. A number of interesting results emerged, and can be summarised in the following key points (for fuller details, see Krasnik *et al.*, 1990). First, there was a tendency for the GPs to change to a greater extent in the short run than in the longer run. This would fit with the idea that they were aiming for a 'target income' (which might simply have been their former income). For fear in the short run of falling short of that former income level with the new remuneration system, they 'overshot', then realising this, eased off and did a bit less. Second, while there was something of a shift in the mix of types of contact with patients, the overall picture was one of little change. Third, substantial change occurred in what the doctors did to the patients once the patients got to the surgery. There is a very large increase in activity per patient for these services which attracted extra fees (removal of warts, etc.) in addition to consultation fees. Further, there were falls of what seem really very large proportions in onward referrals to specialists and hospital. As Table 9.3 indicates, the referrals to specialists fell in comparison with the control by a quarter and to hospital by one third.

These last figures are quite extraordinary. Moving from a capitation system to a part-capitation part-FFS system got doctors to reduce their referrals to specialists by one in four and to hospitals by one in three! There clearly is considerable discretion on the part of GPs in how they act and remuneration systems can push them to go one way or another in how they treat their patients and whether they treat them themselves or refer them on in the system.

Table 9.2   Estimated changes in number of contacts per 1,000 enlisted patients in March and November 1988 compared with that in March 1987 in Copenhagen City (95 per cent confidence interval) and change in Copenhagen County, by type of contact.

Type of contact	March 1987	Copenhagen City		Copenhagen County	
		March 1988	November 1988	March 1988	November 1988
Face-to-face consultations	100	112.7 (106.8 to 118.8)	104.4 (98.9 to 110.2)	105.5	104.9
Consultations by telephone	100	118.6 (108.5 to 129.7)	115.4 (105.5 to 126.3)	108.4	104.0
Renewal of prescriptions	100	82.5 (68.4 to 99.7)	65.2 (53.2 to 79.9)	91.5	92.6
Total	100	111.7 (106.4 to 117.4)	104.2 (99.1 to 109.6)	106.0	104.0

Table 9.3 Estimated changes in number of activities per 1,000 enlisted patients in March and November 1988 compared with that in March 1987 in Copenhagen City (95 per cent confidence interval) and change in Copenhagen County, by type of activity.

Type of activity	March 1987	Copenhagen City		Copenhagen County	
		March 1988	November 1988	March 1988	November 1988
Diagnostic services	100	138.1 (118.7 to 160.5)	159.5 (137.8 to 184.7)	105.3	107.6
Curative services	100	194.6 (152.2 to 248.9)	194.8 (152.3 to 249.2)	106.0	115.0
Referrals to specialist	100	90.1 (80.7 to 100.6)	77.0 (68.6 to 86.4)	99.4	98.1
Referrals to hospital	100	87.4 (71.1 to 107.5)	68.4 (54.7 to 85.4)	97.1	102.1

It is also clear that if doctors are paid more to do something, then they are more likely to do it. That is not surprising, although again the extent of the influence in the case of the Copenhagen City GPs is noteworthy, with increases well above 50 per cent on an average. What has not been reported previously from this study is that there is also some evidence to indicate that the more the GPs are paid per minute for a particular service (this was not constant across all services), the greater was the increase in the service concerned. (These figures are gross remuneration per minute while net would be the preferred figures to use. However it was not possible to get the net figures. Despite this a relationship did emerge, showing that there was a greater increase in services, the greater the gross amount the GP received per minute.)

It is thus the case that such a change in remuneration can have a quite dramatic effect on the way that GPs carry out their medical practice. There seems nothing wrong ethically in this. It does, however, suggest that the medical model, which is often based on the idea that if the diagnosis is X then the treatment is Y, is perhaps a rather simple interpretation of the way that doctors practise. They are influenced by how well they themselves do out of treating or not treating.

What this means is that we have a very powerful tool of health policy which can get doctors to alter their treatment patterns radically and can get them to alter their referral patterns radically also. While other studies have shown somewhat similar results, at least in directions of change, none has shown that remuneration can affect doctors' behaviour to quite such an extent.

Is the extra servicing of patients after the change in Copenhagen City in any sense 'unethical'? I do not think so, as it is difficult to argue that what they were doing previously was ethical nor that what they were doing after was actually against the best interests of the patients. Indeed, it may have been more in the interests of patients. Is it more efficient? We do not know because we do not know enough about what constitutes efficient practice in general practice. Was it more in line with the objectives of the general practitioner service in Copenhagen City? We do not know that either because we do not know what the objectives are in these terms. Does it represent a better mix in terms of allocative efficiency in that it altered the mix between GP, specialist and hospital? We do not know because no one has worked out properly what the most efficient mix is.

Another feature of this study that is worthy of note is that the reason for the change in Copenhagen City was that the GPs there felt that, in terms of income, they were falling behind their FFS counterparts in the rest of the country. They were thus wanting to earn more and so were in a position to do so after the change. To change the remuneration system elsewhere, but where this background did not apply, might well have yielded different results. We cannot tell how much the results are due to the circumstances leading up to the change.

Second, while the results are in line with the idea of a target income for the GPs, they are in line with other possible hypotheses as well. Consequently, I do not think that too much should be made of that point. However, the appearance of being risk-averse in terms of wishing to avoid falling below the former level of income seems a very likely explanation of the way in which servicing of patients rose initially, but then to some extent fell back a little. The implications of this are perhaps more important for research than for policy in that other similar studies in the future might again want to have two after-periods to study and not just one.

Third, the results suggest that supplier-induced demand may have been present. However, it could be that the change in remuneration simply led to doctors being more willing to supply services and that this is a standard market response on the supply side to the raising of prices. (Other things being equal, if the price of a commodity goes up, more of it will be provided on the market.)

It is also relevant to note that, by and large, the GPs did not induce patients but they increased the servicing of the patients. Pertinent to this issue is that the patients, apart from the time costs, did not have to pay any more for these extra services once they were at the surgery. So the extra services provided are principally based on extra remuneration for the doctors and are little affected or constrained by any extra costs falling on the patients.

Given the way that doctors reacted to the changed remuneration and the fact that they are less well placed to induce patients than to induce services for those patients who present anyway suggests that the notion of supplier-induced demand (SID) is a misnomer and that what there is here is supplier-induced *need* (SIN). In fact, it is one of the other advantages of this particular study that it allows a separation of patient inducement from service inducement. This latter seems much more likely in reality and is rather different from SID.

What this also shows, perhaps, is that the whole concept of need, which so often in the medical and epidemiological literature takes on the appearance of being some wholly objective measurable entity, is in practice highly subjective and is a function *inter alia* of how we pay our doctors. Not that I think there is anything wrong with that, but it does cast doubt on the idea that need is 'out there' waiting to be measured!

I would suggest that this adds a further nail to the coffin of the 'needs assessors' (as discussed in Chapter 3).

I do not mean to suggest that there is no evidence on paying doctors other than the Copenhagen study (for this, see Donaldson and Gerard, 1989; and Hemenway *et al.*, 1990). Nor do I want to imply that doctors are only interested in money. In a study I conducted with a colleague in Norway we concluded (Kristiansen and Mooney, 1993) that 'doctor density and turnover appear to be at least as important as the nature of the remuneration system' in influencing practice patterns. Further, we claimed that 'all these factors are weak when compared with the influence of the age and sex of the patient, referrals and medical procedures . . . [and] that the medical problem at hand has a greater influence on clinical practice than organisational factors.' As a potential patient, I think that that is rather reassuring!

It is clear, however, that doctors can be influenced by how they are paid and, given the changes recorded in their behaviour in the Copenhagen study, such changes can be substantial. Using the remuneration system to modify doctors' behaviour is not necessarily unethical, and indeed is unlikely to be so. This is especially so when it is recognised that whatever system of remuneration is in place, it says something about the pattern of incentives that a health service, even if unwittingly, wants doctors to face. To attempt wittingly to influence what doctors do does not affect the ethics of such payment systems.

There does seem to be some misunderstanding of the role of ethics at this level. It is not that ethics dictates to doctors what they do in the sense that there is only one, uniquely correct way of treating a particular patient or problem. Ethics is better seen as dictating – if it dictates at all – what doctors are *not* to do rather than what they are to do. This means in practice that there is a *range* – and often a wide range – of responses from doctors to a particular problem, and all the responses in that range are ethical. It also follows that the fact that doctors can be persuaded to do different things when faced with different remuneration for their activities is not unethical, provided, of course, that the incentives are such that they do not tempt them outside that ethical range.

Is there any justification for concern about FFS medicine? Culyer (1991) for example has suggested that there is scope for being relieved that the NHS reforms in the United Kingdom did not go down the road of FFS medicine. Here, however, I am recommending FFS medicine as at least one way of providing the sort of incentive structure to get doctors to practise more efficiently. My reasoning at this level is that FFS medicine *per se* is not 'bad' even if it is the case that it can provide incentives for inefficiency and perhaps 'overservicing'. Yet these are difficult judgements to make against a background where there is little evidence to show what efficient care is or what optimal servicing levels are. Ignoring that, however, it might still be argued in some quarters that any structure of incentives will get doctors to do more than they would under a capitation or salaried system.

This does not follow. Much will depend on what it is that doctors are contracted to do for their remuneration, whatever form that takes. Whatever the system of payment there is some sort of incentive structure underlying it. That is just as true of capitation and salary as it is for FFS (even if it may well be that the last will be more predictable in its effects).

Another point that emerges from the Copenhagen study is relevant here. Within FFS there are various possible structures of fees. Much emphasis seems to be given to the *level* of fees but not so much to that of structure. Gray (1980), for example, found that the fee structure for Scottish dentists was time neutral in the sense that they were paid approximately the same per minute whatever service they were providing. In the Copenhagen GP structure of remuneration it was clear that the remuneration per minute varied substantially (approximately tenfold) depending on what the doctor was doing.

This variation is very likely to have an effect on how doctors practise. Indeed, in devising the structure of fees one would like to think that this is recognised. Thus in the case of the Scottish dentists we can assume that the intent was that the fee schedule was neutral and that the policy makers had no wish to influence what dentists did beyond specifying the range of treatments which were to be included in the fee schedule. Where, however, the fee schedule is not neutral with respect to time, it ought to be the case that the policy makers have thought this through and decided that some treatments are to be given higher priority than others and consequently have higher financial rewards attached to them per minute spent on them. (In the case of Copenhagen it was clear that that was *not* done, and that the financial reward per minute had not been thought through in this way.)

As a result of this variation in the fees paid in Copenhagen, as indicated above, there is an indication that those services for which the reward per minute was high increased more than for those where it was low. Also, although the effect was not statistically significant, for those services where the reward per minute was the lowest, the level of provision of service seems actually to have *fallen* – and this despite the fact that these services now attracted a fee for the doctor which they had not previously.

The explanation for such a phenomenon is simple and indeed such behaviour is to be expected. Given now (and in this respect the past does not matter) the choice of spending time on some activity which attracts, say $10 per minute or one that attracts $1 per minute, *ceteris paribus*, most of us would opt for the activity that provided the higher reward. When there was no fee for either service we would be neutral in terms of which we did. Now the opportunity cost of the low (but positive) fee service is high and we are thus less likely to perform that service. Consequently, this example shows that the *structure* of fees is crucial in determining what the effect will be on levels of provision of different services and that, provided there is a sufficient range of rewards per minute, it may be possible to use a structure of fees in such a way that some services are provided at a higher level and that some are provided at a lower level than would be the case under a salaried or capitation structure of remuneration. It is the opportunity cost that matters, not the fact that fees are positive *per se*.

There is too little recognition of this point in the health economics literature. Yet in the principal agent literature in economics more generally (see, for example, Ryan, 1992) the issue of the complexity of fee structures is a major one. Trying to get agents to act in a way that gives the principal what he or she wants is difficult, and devising fee structures to deliver is recognised as being very complicated. Yet the thinking there has not been transferred to the health economics literature, where we can still have blunderbuss statements about the rights and wrongs of FFS as a system. There is scope for a lot of research here to look more closely at this issue and in particular to examine situations where it is not just that the doctor is acting as the agent for the patient but also where he or she performs that role on behalf of the funders.

Research on this topic can be difficult to set up. I have worked on GP remuneration in Norway as well as Denmark (see, for example, Kristiansen and Mooney, 1993). The Norwegian work has been difficult because of the research base with which we had to work. There GPs in certain parts of the country can choose whether to be paid on a salaried basis or FFS. Research has looked at how the GPs work under these two systems. The results, however, always have to be qualified in that there may well be variations across the regions under investigation or among the GPs involved, which would explain in part or in whole variations which otherwise might be ascribed to the different remuneration systems. While statistical techniques can help to sort out the strengths of the various factors at work, the beauty of the Copenhagen study was that it was a before and after study of a 'captive' group of GPs working with the same groups of patients and in the same geographical location, admittedly over two different time periods but with a good control available to allow for changes over time. To that extent we were lucky to be able to use that particular research base and hence research design in Denmark. Yet we almost missed the boat in this study and the reason is worth noting.

We realised in late 1986/early 1987 that as a result of a dispute in Copenhagen between the GPs and their employers there was the possibility of looking at the effects of a likely change in the way that GPs were paid. Yet trying to get hold of funds quickly to allow the study to be done, especially to cover the 'before' period, proved difficult. There was nowhere to go in the Danish system to secure funding for such 'opportunistic' research quickly. We managed as a result of the considerable efforts of two of the team but it was difficult, one might say needlessly so. There is thus another lesson from the Copenhagen study here but this time for funders. Try if possible to have a 'contingency fund' to meet the demands that might suddenly arise from such opportunistic research and have a mechanism available to have these funds tapped quickly (for example, without having the whole committee meeting to make the decision). There have to be occasions in health services research where such funds are needed for opportunistic research and where, if the mechanism is not there to have such funding made available fast, good research opportunities will go begging.

What is of much greater concern and at a policy level is that while we know we can influence what doctors do by changing the financial and non-financial incentives they face, there is (1) too little recognition of this as a policy tool in health care; (2) too little information about just what the impact of different incentive and remuneration systems is on doctors' behaviour; and (3) too little thought given to trying to decide what societies want their doctors to do anyway!

I have sought to emphasise in this book that if we cannot get doctors to be efficient, we cannot hope to have efficient health services. Yet here in doctor remuneration we have a potentially very good tool to influence doctors in the direction of practising more efficiently. It can also help to improve their ways of practising and to get done in primary care what is most efficiently done there and have doctors refer patients on in the system when that is the efficient thing to do. Yet we lack understanding of the influence of this tool and we lack knowledge of what is efficient practice. There is scope for doing better here!

Non-paying patients

Several arguments can be put forward for patient payments. However few stand up to any sort of serious investigation. Here I want to examine one of the main arguments that has been advanced – the question of so-called 'moral hazard' – and to indicate why I think it is at best problematical. I will also examine more briefly some of the other arguments for and against patient payment.

One of the key arguments advanced in favour of patient payment is that associated with what is called 'moral hazard', which was first defined by Drèze (1961). Subsidised prices lead to consumer moral hazard which in turn results in a welfare loss because consumers overconsume. This is very much a neoclassical argument. The best price for a market is the clearing price where demand and supply come into equilibrium. If such market prices are subsidised, then consumers will consume more than would otherwise be the case. In the context of car repairs, for example, it is argued that where insurance applies, drivers may drive less carefully than they otherwise would as they will not have to meet the full cost of any accident they then incur; and second, the repairers may do more work than is necessary (and a more expensive job) than they would if the driver had to meet the full cost of the repair.

> Suppose that I wish to evaluate the subjective probability attached by Mr X to the contingency that his car be stolen within a year. What would happen if I were to offer Mr X a prize of say, one million francs, leaving it up to him to choose whether the prize be staked on the theft of his car within a year, or on the opposite contingency? Clearly the alternative chosen by Mr X will exert a definite influence on the caution with which he uses his car, and it will be difficult for me to draw from this experiment any conclusion whatever regarding the probability which Mr X did attach to the possible theft of his car before he accepted the wager. (Drèze, 1961)

It has been suggested (McGuire *et al.*, 1989) that the concept of moral hazard, which in the health economics literature is particularly associated with the name of Mark Pauly (1968), is 'a perfect example of squeezing the analysis of health care into the neoclassical paradigm'. The argument – the neoclassical argument – for moral hazard runs as follows. The conventional (neoclassical) demand curve on which the theory of moral hazard rests assumes a rational, informed consumer. Such a consumer, when faced with competitive market prices, will make efficient choices and in such a way as to maximise her own utility given income and other constraints. Faced with prices below that level, then *ceteris paribus* the consumer will consume 'too much' of that commodity. What is also relevant but is less often emphasised is that this will in turn lead to 'underconsumption' of other commodities, since we have to assume that the consumer has a fixed income. As a result of the 'overconsumption' of one commodity and the 'undercon-sumption' of others, there is a so-called welfare loss – the consumer is worse off than she need be and would be if market prices prevailed throughout.

The question here is: how valid is this (essentially Pauly's) interpretation of moral hazard (Pauly, 1968) in a world where conventional i.e. neoclassical, demand theory may not apply? As Pauly (1986) states in a later article: 'The framework for virtually all the empirical work on insurance effects on demand for medical care has been the very simple model of insurance coverage of a homogeneous medical service.' And he adds: 'In such a model, insurance cuts the use price and thereby increases the physical quantity of services used.' But he adds that it is clear that 'virtually every medical service has a qualitative as well as a quantitative dimension.' He also highlights the fact that very little evidence exists on the qualitative effects of moral hazard.

Within the context of conventional demand theory there are some problems here. Thus, when price is below the full market price, in the standard view of moral hazard, 'too much' health care is consumed and too little preventive action taken. The first of these points assumes simply a movement down the demand curve for the homogeneous commodity health care. Another possible effect, however, is that, given that the commodity health care is not homogeneous, there may be a shift in the demand curve, for example, to some lower quality form of care. Indeed, it may be that the shift is to a higher level of quality. If consumers do not have to meet the true price of their consumption, they may 'demand' higher quality care if it does not attract a higher price. What forms of health care (in terms of quality) will be supplied in markets subject to moral hazard is less than clear, i.e. it is not immediately predictable whether suppliers will offer higher or lower or the same quality of care. If left to the suppliers they might well opt for higher quality or – what might be a more accurate description – more intensive, more technological care. If, however, the consumer cannot judge quality in this market, there could be a lowering of quality as consumers, not having to pay the full market price, lose some of their perceived property rights over the monitoring of quality. (Note that this explanation is a non-neoclassical one.)

Pauly (1986) sees the quality issue in another perspective, however – essentially a supply-side perspective:

> The reason why an individual hospital may choose to provide the same level of service intensity or quality to all buyers, even if some of them might prefer different levels, is the presence of fixed costs associated with supplying each level of product variety. In some sense, the hospital then responds to the average desired level of product quality; if the desired level is determined primarily by insurance coverage, it responds to the average

(or perhaps the modal) level of coverage of demanders in its market. But there may be a much simpler explanation here: the consumer cannot judge or at least has great difficulty in doing so.

Perhaps the most important issue of all is the question of a supply-side response. In neoclassical economics it is taken as given that supply and demand are independent. In health care, given the nature of the commodity involved, this independence appears to break down.

Let us remind ourselves of some of the issues here, quoting from Barr (1987):

> There are other areas (i.e. other than health care) in which the consumer knows little and has to rely on the supplier for information (e.g. hi-fi, used cars). But in these cases it is usually possible to buy information (e.g. consumer magazines, or a report by the Automobile Association [a UK non-profit making organisation which is financed by motorists' subscriptions]), and legislation offers increasing consumer protection. With medical care the costs of mistaken choice are usually greater and less reversible than with most other commodities; an individual generally does not have time to shop around if his condition is acute; doctors are frequently reluctant to offer assessments of colleagues; and consumers frequently lack the information to weigh one doctor's advice against another's. Finally, health and health care have strongly emotive connotations, e.g. ignorance may in part be a consequence of fear, superstition, etc.

Barr at the same time draws attention to the fact that it has been suggested in the United Kingdom that there should be a consumer magazine about medicine, which might be called *Which Doctor?*. It is an interesting idea and it might be useful to speculate over what the contents might include; and how best the information might be obtained.

With respect to the supply-side response, it would seem that something of a question mark has to be placed over the 'conventional' moral hazard concept and interpretation. The implication of the conventional approach is that the demand curve around which or down which moral hazard is defined is the conventional demand curve of the informed, rational consumer. In this context let me quote from the Canadian health economist trio, Barer, Evans and Stoddart (1979) from their classic work on patient payment *Controlling Health Care Costs by Direct Charges to Patients: Snare or Delusion?*

> the influence of economists in helping to keep the direct charge concept alive and well in the United States should not be underestimated. It is well known that gentle massaging of relatively straightforward economic models can yield predictions of an adverse impact of direct charges on total health

care expenditures. Furthermore, with the assumption [which underlies most of the writings on moral hazard] that patients are fully informed consumers, those same models will also tell us that the least efficacious services will be those first deterred. But demand theory applied in this manner is devoid of any consideration of need, agency relationships, and the reasons for their importance in this market. While convenient and conventional, it may also be misleading . . . .. The persistence with which economists return to the fully informed sovereign consumer model in studying health care may have psychological roots: it may also reflect the fine old economic concept of comparative advantage. Economists are much more adept at manipulating this model than are other health care analysts; conversely many of them are much less well informed about the institutional structure of health care delivery. It shows.

(It may be worth stressing that this was written by economists.)

I am not trying to argue that moral hazard does not exist. Rather, I simply want to caution against the assumption that the welfare loss associated with moral hazard can be accurately measured by the conventional measure of excess demand associated with operating in the health care market at a lower price than that associated with the market equilibrium price. Put more bluntly: since in many and perhaps most health care transactions we do not know where the fully informed consumer's demand curve lies, how can the conventional measure of welfare loss associated with excess demand be measured? And if we could identify the ill-informed consumer's (i.e. the more real world) demand curve, and if we could then estimate the welfare loss of moral hazard from that curve, what relationship might that then bear to the 'true' welfare loss? There is some muddled thinking on this issue.

One other relevant aspect relates more directly to the agency relationship (see Chapter 6). Arrow (1986), in his consideration of the principal–agent relation, proposes that there are two types of problem: hidden action and hidden information. He suggests that more normally in the literature these are referred to as moral hazard and adverse selection, respectively. Adverse selection, however, we normally think of as arising with insurance. Because there is (normally) heterogeneity of risk in the insured population, if all are charged the same premium, then as compared with what would be optimal (if differentiation by risk were feasible and if equity were not a consideration) high-risk cases will consume too much and low-risk cases too little. It is likely then that low-risk cases will wish to insure only alongside other low-risk cases and at a low premium, thereby leaving higher-risk cases with higher premiums. (This phenomenon is closely associated with that of 'cream-skimming', where insurers seek to 'cream off' the good risks where premiums are likely to be greater than the expected costs of care and attempt to drop the poor risk people whose premiums are less likely to cover their expected costs of care.)

But there is another facet of this 'hidden information' phenomenon that is relevant to health care and which would not be encapsulated in the normal usage of the term 'adverse selection'. To bring this feature out Arrow (1986) uses the example of optimal income taxation. Here any income tax creates distortion between income and leisure. However, he states: 'This deficiency could in principle be overcome completely if the social price of leisure (i.e. the productivity or wage rate of the individual) were observable. But in general, this information is available to the taxpayer but not to the government.'

In the context of health care the missing information to the government or health care agency is the social price of health. However, this may be known only 'fuzzily' to the individual patient (at least relatively *vis-à-vis* his or her knowledge of the income/leisure trade-off as in Arrow's example) and only with difficulty (and thereby dependent on effort and incentives to find out) to the doctor agent.

What this suggests is the possibility that there are two problems. First, as indicated, the demand curve on which the welfare loss of moral hazard would normally be calculated cannot be considered to be that of the conventional, fully informed consumer. Second, because of the doctor's potential role in reducing – or failing to reduce – the 'fuzziness' experienced by the consumer in interpreting the link between health care consumption and health, the doctor can influence the consumer's perception of the commodity health care. In other words, the doctor not only has the possibility of influencing the weights attached to the good's characteristics but can also actually influence the patient in his/her interpretation of which characteristics are present and without the principal-patient's being able to monitor the agent-doctor's behaviour in this context. (This in one sense goes back to the question of what the arguments are in the patient's utility function, as discussed in Chapter 2. It goes further, however, in the sense of considering the question of monitoring the amount of effort by the doctor in attempting first, to find out what is in the patient's utility function; and second, to help the patient to maximise whatever it is that is there.)

Even Pauly (1986) seems to have some doubts about the problems of quality and moral hazard. He states:

> if insurance displays qualitative moral hazard but the market for the service to which the moral hazard applies is not the simple perfectly competitive, homogeneous product case, then an ordinary demand elasticity (of quantity) will not be a satisfactory summary of the impact of insurance coverage on total expenditures.

I would want to add that it will not provide a satisfactory basis for estimating the welfare loss either.

It is worth noting that in this same article, Pauly (1986) does address questions of supply-side response. At that time, however, he was suggesting 'the existence of demand creation remains an open question' and, second, that 'there is strong evidence that consumer information matters for the market.' It is also possible that where patients are not otherwise informed about quality of care, a higher fee (to attend a specialist direct) rather than a lower one (for a GP consultation) can be the only 'quality' signal available to the poorly informed patient, which could result in increased demand for the higher priced service (see Monroe and Krishman, 1984). There is an example of this type of response in Iceland in 1985.

In an FFS system, the lack of a supply-side response also requires that doctors passively accept that, *ceteris paribus*, higher patient fees will result in their incomes falling. Given the evidence (Rice and Labelle, 1989; Rice, 1983) both on supplier induction and on the target income hypothesis, such doctor passivity seems unlikely. It is clearly more likely in salaried or capitation systems. Note also that the health effects are also potentially of concern. If doctors are able to induce demand for those who do visit, the induced care is likely to be less effective than that cut off by the patient payment. However, such a hypothesis would need to be subjected to empirical analysis and the results would probably be quite specific to the local circumstances.

What the impact of patient payment on health service expenditure will be in these circumstances is much more difficult to predict than the simple conventional demand approach suggests. Clearly, the RAND experiment (as reported by Manning *et al.*, 1987), which constitutes the biggest experiment on patient payments ever undertaken, is particularly germane – or at least so it seems at first. The experiment was set up in the United States and ran from 1974 to 1982.

While there were a number of facets to it, in the context of the discussion here the key elements were as follows. Over 2,000 families were randomly allocated to fourteen different insurance plans, which varied *inter alia* in terms of the extent of patient payment. The influence of the supply-side response was assumed to be negligible because no participating doctor had more than a small proportion of his or her patients covered by the experiment. As McGuire *et al.* (1989) state: 'The results tend to confirm the view that consumption is dependent upon the form of insurance coverage and specifically that consumption increases as out-of-pocket expenses decrease.' For example, for adults, cost sharing resulted in a more than 30 per cent decrease in outpatient visits, and hospitalisation admissions fell by about the same proportion. Care is needed, however, in interpreting these results, especially as there have to be some reservations about the study design and the generalisability of the results to other settings – a point I will return to below.

More and/or better consumer information could, of course, help to improve efficiency in health care. This is dealt with at greater length in Chapter 10, where competition is discussed.

A number of points arise from this. First, whatever is done about consumer information in health care, it is difficult to accept that we can ever talk in general about conventional demand curves for (most forms of) health care. It is common for economists at this point to suggest that much of primary care may be an exception to this. I would say some, rather than much, and given the discussion of the Copenhagen study presented earlier in this chapter, the notion of conventional demand may be restricted not just to first visits *per se* but to the attending. In other words, patients make (largely) sovereign decisions about attending (or calling in) a doctor at the start of an episode of illness. Beyond that however (i.e. not beyond the first visit but beyond getting to the doctor) conventional demand ceases to retain its full meaning. We are not dealing with an independent, rational informed consumer. We are faced with something akin to SIN – supplier-induced *need*.

Second, the evidence that doctors can influence the use of health care through the patient – whether this is to be deemed 'conventional SID', however, is another matter (as I argue in Chapter 10) – is now so strong that it ceases to be reasonable to argue that there is still a question mark over its existence, only over its form and extent.

Third, there can be little doubt that moral hazard does exist. If any commodity is sold below its full market price, then the logic of demand theory points to excess consumption of that commodity and consequently less than optimal demand of at least some other commodities. The problem is whether conventional analysis provides an appropriate framework for predicting the impact on behaviour, expenditures and welfare as a result of the existence of moral hazard. Given the nature of 'demand' in the health care 'market', that seems unlikely.

In this context let me quote Evans (1984). He suggests that analyses of moral hazard tend to 'leave out of account . . . any other peculiarities, intrinsic or derived, of the commodity "health care" itself.' He continues:

the fact that health status depends, in a technical way, on health care, simultaneously demolishes the basis for the assumption that consumers are, in fact, informed. If they are not, and their ignorance is remedied by provider-supplied information, then 'the demand curve' . . . may not exist as a stable, negative relationship between prices paid by users and quantities consumed. And even if it does exist, it loses its normative significance as a guide to 'appropriate' resource allocation.

As so often, I think Bob Evans gets right to the heart of things with these comments!

Fourth, it is to be noted that it is not just consumers who are subject to moral hazard in health care; so also are doctors, in the sense that they supply treatments, diagnostic tests, etc., often without even approximate knowledge of the costs of doing so. Indeed, while the great majority of the literature on moral hazard concentrates on consumers it may well be that supply-side moral hazard is at least as serious a problem. (For a good account of producer moral hazard, see Donaldson and Gerard, 1993.) As Evans (1984) remarks in his extension of moral hazard problems to the supply side:

> The potential sources of 'moral hazard' in response to insurance coverage
> include independent forms of supplier behaviour – raising prices or changing
> recommendations about care use . . .. Possessing the . . . power to
> influence patients' utilization patterns directly, providers can, and do, shift
> the demand curve, behaviour it is difficult or impossible to control directly
> in a framework of competitive, private insurance plans dealing with
> suppliers at arm's length . . . the longer term health care cost experience of
> the United States over the last thirty years suggests that present levels of
> insurance coverage in that country . . . are sufficient to permit 'moral
> hazard' on the supply side to generate steadily escalating prices and levels of
> utilization.

Against this background it is clear that interpretation of the results of any studies on patient payment can be difficult and complex. Certainly, the rather naive attitude of many politicians and policy makers to patient payment is frequently unhelpful. This seems often to convert the neoclassical conventional demand analysis discussed above into the notion that higher prices will lead to the reduction of low-valued (by consumers) forms of care, with a subsequent fall in health care costs as this 'trivial' utilisation stops, or at least falls.

Whether what is of 'low value' to the consumer is 'trivial' has to be a matter of some debate. A study in Swaziland (Yoder, 1989), for example, showed that user fees did reduce utilisation, by some 17 per cent. The author states, however: 'The hope that the 17% fewer patient visits would consist primarily of minor ailments or self-limiting diseases is not supported by the data [in the study]. The decreases in immunizations and treatment for diarrhoeal and sexually transmitted diseases suggest that the "wrong people" have left the system.' This is a particularly interesting finding and seems to contradict at least some of the conventional wisdom in this area, especially with respect to financing health care in developing countries. Thus the World Bank issued 'An Agenda for Reform' on financing health services in developing countries (Akin *et al.*, 1987). One of the four key recommendations was to charge users of government health facilities, especially for drugs and curative care. The authors state: 'This will increase the resources available to the government health sector, allow more funding on underfunded programs, encourage better quality and more efficiency, and increase access for the poor.' They add that differential fees should be used to protect the poor, and indeed that the poor 'should be the major beneficiaries of expanding resources for and improved efficiency in the government sector'.

This is somewhat controversial. In justifying it Akin *et al.* (1987) state that

> the more common approach to health care in developing countries has been to treat it as a right of the citizenry and to attempt to provide free services for everyone. This approach does not usually work. It prevents the government health system from collecting revenues that many patients are both able and willing to pay.

As Yoder (1989) counters:

> User fees typically are justified on the grounds that people are willing and able to pay for health services. Evidence in support of this assumption generally derives from household or aggregate expenditure surveys . . . or from attitude surveys in which people are asked how much they would be willing to pay for a particular service . . .

So is the World Bank right to advocate patient charges? Whatever the arguments for and against patient charges, they apply equally in developing and developed countries with one exception. Where insurance and tax systems are not well developed, it may be difficult to finance health services in any way other than user charges. What has to be crucial in any policy in developing countries on user charges is the ability of the system to cross subsidise from rich sick to poor sick – certainly on equity grounds, but probably also on efficiency grounds.

Clearly, the RAND results, as reported by Manning *et al.* (1987) and as reported briefly above, may be relevant to the issue of the actual effects of patient payments. But reservations about the relevance of RAND in the real world are pertinent.

The underlying model in RAND is based very intentionally on conventional demand theory and deliberately attempts to restrict the supply-side response, i.e. to keep doctors passive. This is because the spread of the patients in the study across different doctors was such that no doctor had many patients and consequently any supply-side response was minimised. While this appears to be a deliberate aim of the study designers, it does mean that the effects estimated by Manning *et al.* are not likely to be repeated elsewhere in any real-world situation – at least if one accepts the high probability of non-passive doctors when faced with the prospect of income changes, especially in a downward direction. As Evans (1984) suggests, the results of the RAND experiment 'give no information at all about what the effects would be of a general program of increased charges to patients which would (if it affected use) lower each provider's income and workload. The experimental results, by design, cannot be generalized.' Given that, one could, if one were so inclined, question whether the RAND experiment was worth the very substantial cost involved.

What of the other arguments for patient payments? I will consider these only briefly as I think they are of less importance than is moral hazard and issues related to that phenomenon.

First, patient payments can lead to a reduction in health service costs. If this is an objective of health care, then patient payments do represent one instrument which can help to achieve this goal. They can do so in two ways. First, they can result in fewer patients using the priced service, for example in presenting prescriptions to a chemist for take-up and hence payment. Second, they can reduce expenditure through raising revenue. Thus prescription charges raise revenue for the health service, thereby either reducing overall expenditure on the health service or allowing spending elsewhere in the service at a higher level. Charges to patients can mean fewer patients and also a shift of cost bearing from the health service to the patients.

Whether this is sensible is another matter and, even if it were, the fact that patient payments can result in lower health service costs does not mean that that is necessarily the best way to achieve such savings. From an economic point of view the concern ought to be with efficiency and equity and not cost saving. Patient payments will have an impact on efficiency but just what that impact will be is less than clear. If they result in a reduction in, for example, trivial cases presenting to GPs, thereby allowing GPs to concentrate more of their time and resources generally on cases for which they can do more good, this will result in increased efficiency. However, as discussed above, the question of what constitutes trivia is in the hands of the patients, who do not seem the best judges of what is trivial in health terms. Consequently, if the goal is to increase efficiency by trying to get doctors to spend more time on cases which will respond to their efforts, then a better policy would seem to involve one which allowed the doctor to form the judgement of what is trivial and what is not. More patient education in what sorts of problem are likely to respond to GPs' treatments and what are not might also help to promote efficient resource use at this level. To use patient payments to serve this purpose seems at best too crude and at worst inappropriate as a policy instrument. Patient payments, unless accompanied by a rather precise information base to prevent it and a structure of fees to take account of the differential effects of different levels of payments according to income (and which would quickly become costly to administer), are likely to have adverse effects on the pursuit of the goal of equity across different socio-economic groups.

Some of the gains that are attributed (even if falsely) to patient payments in this context may be obtained – and without such severe side effects – through making patients aware of the costs of treatment of different forms without actually having them make payments for the treatment. Such information might be included in the education of patients in health service use.

It would also be possible to use patient payments to promote allocative efficiency by having differential payments for different types of treatment. Payments might be set in such a way as to try to influence the use of health services to reflect relative social priorities for different forms of care. This does occur already in some health services, in that some groups, such as pregnant women, may be exempt from patient charges. But in principle it would be possible to devise a structure of fees – both positive and negative – to try to influence health service use in such a way as to promote more allocatively efficient resource use in health care.

The potential for success of such an approach appears not to have been examined, perhaps because it would quickly become very complicated to administer. More importantly, there are again stronger arguments in favour of other policies to promote allocative efficiency, particularly using budget allocations in health care and operating on incentives for the doctors rather than for the patients – yet again.

On equity grounds patient payments would clearly have adverse effects unless again they were set in such a way as to account for variations in income across populations. However, such variations seldom are taken into account and even less frequently with any degree of refinement. Exempting the poor is often the extent of any differential that is applied, or having a maximum payment over a period of, say, a year. Consequently, in practice, patient payments tend to be inequitable.

Paying doctors and paying patients

Is there some combination of patient payments and payment of doctors that can be used as a policy tool to promote efficiency in health care and, indeed, equity? Taking the latter first, it will be clear from what has been said earlier in this chapter that the usefulness of patient payments, as normally conceived, to promote equity in health care is limited and frequently will be adverse. In terms of patients and potential patients with different incomes, if an objective of health care is to provide health or to allow use of or access to health care irrespective of income, then patient payments are very likely to come in the way of such a goal. There is no real argument against such a view.

There may be instances, however, where a health care system might want to experiment with 'negative patient payments' in an effort to promote equity. The most obvious form of such payments would be to compensate those who have long distances to travel to services by, for example, paying or subsidising their transport costs and perhaps also their travel time. A health service which supports an objective of equity where equity is defined in terms of equal access may find that the most efficient way of promoting this objective is through paying or subsidising patients' costs in attending. To achieve more equal access by taking services to patients may, on occasion, be very expensive.

The nature of such subsidisation, however, would need to be examined carefully. What is required if equality of access is the equity goal (see Chapter 5) is that patients face the same opportunity cost of using the service. Given that the same money or time cost may have a different opportunity cost to different individuals, determining precisely what the amount of the subsidies would be to equate with such opportunity costs would be difficult in practice. For example, the system would need to distinguish between those who were taking time off work with their incomes protected, those who took time off but lost pay as a result, and those who were not gainfully employed. The relevant costs here are the opportunity costs *to the individual* and not to society. These difficulties in practice, however, are no reason for not experimenting more than has been the case to date with such negative payments to promote equity.

Where the equity goal is equal use or equal health, then there may be a case for using negative patient payments to try to correct 'wrong' or 'inappropriate' preferences for health care on the part of 'underutilisers'. Where use is the dimension of equity, in the sense that the objective is couched in terms of equal use for equal need, then even where access for equal need is achieved, equal use may not follow. This would be the case when individuals had lower preferences for health care than others had. In order to adjust for this, a policy might be put in place not to adjust the preferences of these underutilisers in an upward direction (which is the source of the problem here) but to reduce their costs of use. In this way, while they would be left with their 'deficient' preferences, they could have equal use as compared with those with the same need but whose preferences were not deficient. This is 'positive discrimination' where the underutilisers would be given better access than others, i.e. their costs of using the health care system would be reduced.

There are several ways of doing this, such as taking the services closer to the underutilisers. Thus if there were a social class gradient, it might be that taking services closer to poorer parts of cities – providing clinics for antenatal care in working-class housing estates, for example – would be one way of positively discriminating to raise the use of this group. Another approach would be to provide financial incentives to working-class pregnant women to attend, and these financial incentives would be in essence negative patient payments. However, it is first necessary to accept the definition of equity as being equal use for equal need before going down this road. For many I suspect this is too elitist a definition and consequently positive discrimination of this particular type would not be seen as an appropriate policy instrument.

It is also possible to argue that to achieve equal use for equal need, instead of using negative patient payments for the underutilisers, there could be positive patient payments for the 'overutilisers' or some combination of negative and positive payments. Thus instead of promoting more equal use in an upward direction, such equal use could be at some lower level. It seems likely, given how difficult it would be to achieve it, that if the equity goal were equal health – and equal health irrespective of baseline need – the only practical way of achieving equal health would be to bring the health of the healthy down, rather than through moving the health of the unhealthy up! Yet Culyer (1991), for example, in advocating that equality of health be the equity goal, has argued that this would only be pursued in an upward direction. As I have indicated in Chapter 5, this would mean that the achievement of such a position would be a very long time into the future.

At the level of efficiency there can be an argument for patient payments in some circumstances, perhaps to steer patients away from inefficient use of health services. But the process is a difficult one and would seem better avoided if possible. In Iceland the larger but still small payment that patients had to make to attend a specialist rather than a general practitioner in the 1980s seemed to result in the patients believing, or believing more, that the more expensive doctor was the better doctor. Demand for specialist services was then less constrained than had been thought in advance of the introduction of this differential pricing system.

Where patient payments can be used – even if they remain not the best way to influence the system to deliver efficiency – is where they are a mechanism to influence not only the behaviour of the patients but also the behaviour of the doctors. As mentioned above, where there are patient payments, then the form these take can be better or worse for guiding the system towards more or less efficient resource use. Proportional patient payments (i.e. where the payment is some fraction of the overall cost) can be used to influence the patient to opt for a cheaper drug, for example, and also to influence the doctor to prescribe a cheaper drug when acting as the patient's agent and having a concern not only for the patient's health but also for the patient's income. There is some tentative evidence from Denmark (and intuitively one can see how it comes about) that doctors may be more concerned about costs falling on their patients than those falling on 'the system' or on the service as a whole. Clearly where a charge is a fixed absolute amount (as in the United Kingdom for prescriptions), then the doctor, as the patient's agent, will not be influenced in this way even if as society's agent he or she should still be concerned about the cost to the system.

The Icelanders adopted such a system by indicating for each category of drug that one is the preferred choice in terms of therapeutic value and cost. Backed by a major publicity campaign, a system was introduced whereby the preferred drug was always the cheapest in that category to the patient. The doctor and the patient could decide to choose another drug but if they did, the patient had to pay more. While there are no data on how this system has worked, it is an interesting use of patient payments in the context of the doctor as the patient's agent.

More generally with respect to the use of patient payments or doctor payments, the latter seems the better policy tool for the promotion of efficiency. Doctors do have much more say than patients over how resources are used in health care. Certainly while there may be weak arguments (at the level of moral hazard and/or 'triviality') for patient payments for a first visit to a GP in an episode of illness, there seems little justification for such payment for return visits – at least not when, as is usually the case, it is the doctor who proposes the return visit! It is difficult to see how consumer moral hazard or triviality could apply in these instances.

150   *Key Issues in Health Economics*

References

Akin, J., Birdsall, N. and de Ferranti, D. (1987) *Financing Health Services in Developing Countries, an Agenda for Reform.* The World Bank, Washington, D. C.

Arrow, K. J. (1986) Agency and the market. In K. J. Arrow and M. D. Intrilligator (eds) *Handbook of Mathematical Economics*, vol. III. Elsevier, Amsterdam.

Barer, M. L., Evans, R. G. and Stoddart, G. L. (1979) *Controlling Health Care Costs by Direct Charges to Patients: Snare or delusion?* Ontario Economic Council, Ontario.

Barr, N. (1987) *The Economics of the Welfare State.* Weidenfeld & Nicolson, London.

Culyer, A. J. (1991) Competition and markets in health care: what we know and what we don't. NHS White Paper Occasional Series, Centre for Health Economics, University of York, York.

Donaldson, C. and Gerard, K. (1989) Paying general practitioners: shedding light on the review of health services. *Journal of the Royal College of General Practitioners*, **39**, 114–17.

Donaldson, C. and Gerard, K. (1993) *Financing Health Care.* Macmillan, London.

Drèze, J. H. (1961) Les fondements logique de l'utilité cardinale et de la probabilité-subjective. *La Décision, Colloques Internationaux du CNRs*, Paris.

Evans, R. G. (1984) *Strained Mercy.* Butterworth, Ontario.

Gray, A. M. (1980) The production of dental care in the British National Health Service. HERU Discussion Paper, 08/80, University of Aberdeen, Aberdeen.

Hemenway, D., Killen, A., Cashman, S. B., Parks, C. L. and Bicknell, W. J. (1990) Physicians' responses to financial incentives. *New England Journal of Medicine*, **322**, 1059–63.

Krasnik, A., Groenewegen, P. P., Pedersen, P. A., von Scholten, P., Mooney, G., Gottschau, A., Flierman, H. A. and Damsgaard, M. T. (1990) Changing remuneration systems: effects on activity in general practice. *British Medical Journal*, **300**, 1698–701.

Kristiansen, I. S. and Mooney, G. (1993) Remuneration of GP services: time for more explicit objectives? A review of the systems in five industrialised countries. *Health Policy*, **24**, 203–12.

McGuire, A. J., Henderson, J. B. and Mooney, G. H. (1989) *The Economics of Health Care*, Routledge and Kegan Paul, London.

Manning, W. G., Newhouse, J. P., Guan, N., Keeler, E. B., Leibowitz, A. and Marquis, M. S. (1987) Health insurance and the demand for medical care: evidence from a randomised experiment. *American Economic Review*, **77**, 251-77.

Monroe, K. B. and Krishman, R. (1984) The effect of price on subjective product evaluation. In J. Jacoby and J. Olson (eds), *Consumers of Merchandise and Store Quality.* D. C. Heath, Lexington, Mass.

Pauly, M. V. (1968) The economics of moral hazard: comment. *American Economic Review*, **57**, 231–7.

Pauly, M. V. (1986) Taxation, health insurance, and the market failure in the medical economy. *Journal of Economic Literature*, **XXIV**, 629–75.

Rice, T. (1983) The impact of changing medicare reimbursement rates on physician-induced demand. *Medical Care*, **21**, 8, 803–15.
Rice, T. H. and Labelle, R. J. (1989) Do physicians induce demand for medical services? *Journal of Health Politics, Policy and Law*, **14**, 3, 587–600.
Ryan, M. (1992) The agency relationship in health care; identifying areas for future research. HERU Discussion Paper 02/92, University of Aberdeen, Aberdeen.
Yoder, R. A. (1989) Are people willing and able to pay for health services? *Social Science and Medicine*, **29**, 1, 35–42.

10
Competition and incentives more generally

Introduction

What we are looking for through competition is in essence a set of incentives that will promote efficiency. The questions then become:

1. Does competition promote efficiency?
2. Is competition the best way to promote efficiency?
3. Does competition provide the 'right' set of incentives for efficiency?
4. Does competition provide the 'best' set of incentives for efficiency?

Competition

In addressing these issues there is a need to recognise that the virtues of competition have to be set in a framework of relativities and not judged against some unachievable absolute or golden standard. One of the main criticisms that is often made of public health care systems is that there is a lack of competition and as a result a lack of the kinds of incentive that are present in competitive markets. However, it seems better to argue that public health care systems often have incentive structures in them that seem inappropriate or at best deficient when it comes to the pursuit of the goal of efficiency and often of equity as well. Indeed, while it may be argued that competitive forces may be useful in the promotion of efficiency, there would seem to be general agreement that they are unlikely to promote the objective of equity in health care. Thus even the starting point for considering the virtues of competitive forces – whether the objectives of health care are likely to be promoted through competitive forces – seems immediately to indicate that at least one of the key objectives of most health care systems – equity – is unlikely to be well served by market forces.

Even on the efficiency side of public health care systems there is a need for care. Although it is frequently 'lack of incentives for efficiency' that is the issue, this can quickly be reduced to lack of incentives. Thus a system of retrospective reimbursement of hospitals on a *per diem* basis can be described as lacking incentives whereas in reality the incentive here is clear: there is an incentive to keep beds filled and with not so ill (and therefore not so resource-consuming) patients.

What is normally meant in this area is that there are no or inadequate incentives (1) to keep costs down, or (2) for efficiency. Interestingly – and I will come back to this issue below – there tends to be relatively little written about incentives for increased quality, beyond issues of various forms of quality review, peer review, medical audit, etc.

The other point is that with respect to incentives, economists would normally think of two sets of incentives – one on producers and one on consumers. Yet given the nature of the health care market it is necessary to consider the behaviour of a wider set of actors, including, for example, the funders, and consequently both a wider set of incentives and a greater amount of interaction between different actors.

Additionally, there is a need to address the question of incentives for what. Here there are various possibilities:

1. incentives for increased effectiveness;
2. incentives for decreasing costs;
3. incentives for operational efficiency (combining 1 and 2);
4. incentives for allocative efficiency;
5. incentives for equity; and
6. incentives for change.

A word about the last may be appropriate. Despite the changes currently taking place and planned in health services in various countries, such as the United Kingdom, The Netherlands and New Zealand, the history of health services generally in the last twenty years or so is one which suggests an inherent conservatism. This may be a reflection of many things: the conservatism of the medical profession, the tendency (in most consumer surveys) for patients to express satisfaction with the treatment they have received, the natural 'anti-change' attitudes of most large, bureaucratic organisations. It thus seems that there is a need to consider the last item – incentives for change – rather carefully because if the system won't or can't change, then debating and planning incentives at the other levels will be useless.

One very important and yet very basic aspect of this relates to the setting of objectives. At a clinical level, for example, if doctors do not have a clear, explicit idea of what they are attempting to achieve (beyond some rather general objective of making the patient better), and additionally if there is not a fairly definite, identified road to get there, then setting incentives to get on the right road to achieve objectives is problematical. (The Copenhagen GP study – discussed in Chapter 9 – is a case in point. In making the change in remuneration, the Copenhagen politicians were not clear about what they sought to achieve and, beyond the question of attaining some target income, nor does it seem were the doctors.) It is also far from clear that the objectives built into my listing above (1–5) should be accepted by all health care policy-makers.

Looking at this list with the eyes of an economist and from the perspective of incentives as compared with other policy tools, in health care most of the debate on incentives has been about cutting costs. While this is frequently dressed up in terms of operational efficiency, surprisingly little of the debate encompasses any real notion of increased effectiveness, still less about allocative efficiency and very close to nothing on equity. On incentives for change – systems change – the increased concern in recent years in so many developed countries that health care costs were rising inexorably has perhaps been the greatest incentive for change to try to contain costs. In developing countries, perhaps, the problem has been more how to raise additional funds; but that too has brought pressure to change.

Let us look at the list above. On incentives for effectiveness, one of the most striking aspects of modern medicine, as discussed in Chapter 8, is that there are these very substantial variations in medical practice across countries, but even more striking within countries (Andersen and Mooney, 1990). There are various explanations for the existence of these variations. Without, however, even beginning to consider questions of inefficiency, it has to be the case that some doctors are being more effective than others. There is thus scope for improvements. Despite the strength, breadth and long history of knowledge of these variations, the extent to which policy makers have been concerned to deal with this element of ineffectiveness in any way has been limited. Certainly there has been little evidence of change and little evidence of setting up policies for incentives for change, beyond providing feedback to doctors about the extent of variation. (This policy of feedback may reduce variations but whether it increases effectiveness is not at all apparent.)

This issue can be examined a little more fundamentally through considering the fact that even today there are many clinical trials where results remain measured in terms of some very narrow concept of effectiveness, e.g. mortality or percentage survival after, say, five years. Even if the results of such effectiveness studies were being adequately fed through into medical practice and being picked up quickly and to the same extent by all the relevant doctors, if the concept of effectiveness adopted in the trial is too narrow, the pursued policies might then be ineffective in terms of some broader concept (reflecting, for example, quality of life).

Generally, then, the extent to which incentives exist which are specifically aimed at improving effectiveness remains limited. In the particular context of competition, there is no evidence to suggest that competition decreases the extent of variation in common medical procedures. Certainly, if competition were to lead to the deployment of more resources in the health care system, this might result in increased effectiveness overall (see Chapter 8).

One of the problems with this concern for incentives for effectiveness is that at a general level the extent to which effectiveness or quality of care can be measured is difficult – if, for example, we are considering whether one set of hospitals is more effective than another. The evidence on the impact of competition on quality or effectiveness is very scarce. Certainly, as discussed below, if competition results in reduced length of stay, there is an *a priori* case for arguing that health status at the point of discharge may be reduced. But that would need to be tested empirically as it could well be that the additional stay had a zero effect on the patient's health. Sager *et al.* (1989) report that the greater the competition between hospitals the stronger was the relationship between reduced length of stay and the fall in hospital deaths (due to the 'offloading' of dying cases to nursing homes).

The evidence here on effectiveness is poor, perhaps understandably so. The questions to be answered are difficult: can competition between hospitals reduce costs without affecting outcomes? If it can, what is the greatest reduction in costs possible before outcomes are negatively affected?

What does not appear to have been studied (but I am less clear here) is whether any indicator of quality (effectiveness) increases demand for that service/hospital. This is an assumption which appears to have been built into the NHS reforms. One question it begs in any health care system is who is to judge the quality. It seems unlikely that patients will be well placed to form such judgements, which means that even they may accept that someone else has to perform this role. But who should this be?

It is not immediately clear that competition *per se* is the best form of incentive to increase effectiveness, at least at the hospital level. If competition is to work in any market there has to be some minimum number of competing firms and 'consumers' must have information about the quality of the products. That does not seem like a description of most hospital markets. Other forms of incentives may be preferable or at least needed in addition, such as clinical budgeting plus professional standards reviews (although perhaps more as a regulatory rather than incentive mechanism).

In a sense this pushes us back to consider whether economists really understand the internal behaviour of hospitals or the utility functions of hospital doctors sufficiently to be able to say much about the nature of current incentive structures at the clinical or hospital level. It is perhaps as much or even more the understanding at that level that is needed before we can begin to judge what are the best incentives for promoting effectiveness.

Economists generally have tended to study hospitals at a rather aggregate level, perhaps because the data are more readily available at that level. Yet the driving force in all hospitals lies in the clinical arena and, unless economists can understand that arena better than they currently do, there is little scope for their developing a true perspective on how different forms of incentives might work in the clinical setting of hospitals.

On incentives for decreasing costs, it is worth noting that it is here that there is most evidence on the effect of different mechanisms. That may not be surprising since costs are more easily measured than quality/effectiveness. And it is normally also health service costs, or more narrowly still hospital costs, that get measured. Thus in their review of the effects of competition, Culyer and Posnett (1990) state that they will 'review some more empirical experience in the United States, focusing in particular on the role of competition in *cost containment*' (emphasis added).

In considering paying hospitals there are substantial limitations in the evidence regarding changes in costs as a result of various forms of incentives directed at hospital behaviour.

In recent years perhaps the best-known effort at controlling inpatient hospital costs stems from the so-called 'DRG' initiative in the United States. Within Medicare in that country, in an effort to reduce costs of inpatients in hospitals, the system for paying hospitals was moved from a *per diem* to a case mix basis. Under the former, hospitals were normally paid a flat rate per inpatient day; under the latter payment was by case, with a different fee depending into which category – which diagnosis-related group (DRG) – a patient fell.

There was a clear shift in the structure of incentives with this change. Hospitals no longer have the same incentive to hang on to patients who may be occupying beds cheaply and for whom they receive more than adequate financial compensation on a *per diem* basis. Now that they are paid on a per case basis, i.e. by diagnosis-related group, there is an incentive to move patients through the hospital more quickly, the intention being thereby to reduce hospital inpatient costs.

There is evidence that DRGing in the United States has reduced hospital costs per day and per admission. There is worry also that at least some of this saving has been achieved simply by moving patients out of the inpatient sector to other forms of care not covered by the DRG process. There is also some concern that the quality of care has been reduced. (For a review of this evidence on DRGs generally see Donaldson and Gerard, 1993.)

Three main points need to be made about the DRG initiative. First, despite, on the one hand, the lack of any convincing evidence that DRGing has resulted in an overall reduction in health care costs and, on the other, the existence of some close to convincing evidence that it has led to reduced quality of care, the very considerable extent to which DRGing has become an international health service industry is striking, indeed staggering. So many countries are DRGing or about to DRG! How has this happened? I suspect it is that DRGing is based on what appears in principle to be a convincing argument. Replacing a flat *per diem* rate with a fixed rate per case seems like a good thing. And it may still be the case that it is, even if the actual evidence to date is not persuasive. But in some countries which are busy DRGing it is not a flat *per diem* rate that DRGs are replacing and the case for DRGs – even in principle – then becomes weaker.

Second, DRG costings are average rather than marginal costings. As such, how they are used has to be appraised with the greatest of caution. There are few situations in which average costs are in principle appropriate for use in managing health services. (They may on certain occasions be reasonable approximations to marginal costs but that is a separate issue.)

Third, it is normally the case that the costs associated with each DRG (which are then used in determining the reimbursement levels) are based on what has been happening in the period prior to the introduction of DRGs. This seems odd. The apparent reason to introduce DRGs as the basis for costing is that what has been happening previously with respect to resource use is seen as less than optimal in terms of either efficiency or purely cost. Rather than simply emulate what has been happening, what is wanted is that clinicians and clinical teams use resources in a more efficient way. Yet costing DRGs based on past performances will allow, even promote, inefficient practices to be continued in the future.

What seems to be required is that, first, whatever constitutes efficient practice be determined. Then some mechanism would be introduced to provide the right framework of incentives to encourage such efficient practice in the future. Such a framework might well involve DRGs but using the costings based on whatever it is that is considered to constitute efficient practice, and not practices that are known to be or at the very least thought to be inefficient! (Otherwise why introduce DRGS in the first place?)

What would seem preferable is to give clinicians (or clinical teams) budgets within which to operate and allow them to come to grips with the idea of using these resources as best they can and within this budget. Thereafter, i.e. after they have become used to trying to operate efficiently within this budget, then might be the time to adopt costings of DRGs based on the more efficient practice that will by then have emerged. This clinical budgeting (or resource management initiative as it is called in the NHS in the United Kingdom at present) has not to date been given a sufficient run in this way to determine its true merits.

What of competition more specifically? At least some of the experience here points to competition resulting in increased costs. However, the Californian experience (see Melnick and Zwanziger, 1988) suggests that competition there, in the form of selective contracting, led to a slight fall in the total inpatient costs and in total inpatient days, although with increases in cost per case and cost per day. A large part of the saving in inpatient costs was offset by an increase in outpatient costs. The evidence is not strong and appears to suggest that any possible cost savings may well be small and could be negative.

Again of course, there is a need to take care. Much will depend not just on the incentives within the system but also the ability to cap spending *in toto*. Thus some elements of competition linked to budgeting which can be capped, preferably at various different levels, may be the right mix of incentives to promote cost-cutting. Whether capping plus competition is better in this context than capping minus competition is difficult to judge at present because of lack of evidence.

Certainly it can readily be argued that if competition leads to specialisation within hospitals, this may well help to reduce costs. The question, then, is whether the same specialisation can be achieved without competition.

On operational efficiency – essentially combining effectiveness and costs – it will be clear from what has been said that there is not too much that can be said about competition and operational efficiency. Again, so much would seem to depend on other aspects of the health care environment, especially on capping, clinical budgeting and medical audit.

The question of provision of more and/or better consumer information to help to improve the operational efficiency of health care markets is potentially important. The issue is most frequently raised by those who see the 'market' as the most efficient way of supplying health care but accept, worry about but want to act on improving, the consumer's information problems. Indeed, as Rice and Labelle (1989) state: 'It is hard to object to improved consumer information.'

The question now arises: what is optimal information, given that its obtaining and dissemination are not costless and decisions are needed about its content and presentation? I would argue that it is not information *per se* that is the issue but rather autonomy, which 'implies the ability to govern oneself' (Loewy, 1990).

However, it may be relevant at this juncture to remind readers that the main reason we train medical doctors may be because this is an efficient way of making medical knowledge available to the population as a whole. (That is not an argument against better consumer information, simply a cautionary note.)

An observation from Hibbard and Weeks (1989) on information to consumers is germane. They state: 'While there is general recognition of the need for access to information, there is almost no empiric evidence on if and how consumers will use information in making health care decisions.'

In the light of this, they examined the effect on consumer behaviour of disseminating information on doctors' fees, and concluded that dissemination of this fee information did not lead to reduced health care expenditure. The authors offer three possible explanations for this: 'inadequate financial incentives, incomplete information, and inadequate preparation to make use of this information'.

On the first, the savings to patients through using the information were quite small. The fee for a basic consultation lay between US$18 and US$45, which, with respect to what the patient paid, reduced to a differential of US$5.40.

On the second, Hibbard and Weeks suggest that quality may be the prime factor in consumers' decisions, but that, as Monroe and Krishman (1984) indicate, 'where quality information is unavailable and when consumers have little experience in evaluating the service or product, people will rely on price as a surrogate for quality.'

Their third, and related, explanation is potentially the most interesting for our discussion here, and is worth quoting it at some length.

> The role for the users of health care is that of 'patient'. The patient role is characterised by trust, passivity, compliance, and dependence. To respond to market forces and make decisions based on cost and quality variations requires a different orientation. A consumer, in contrast to a patient, is a questioning, active and informed decision-maker. Consumerism implies at least a partial challenge to physician authority. Recent studies have found that consumerism in health care is relatively rare. Yet, an active informed consumerate [sic] is the cornerstone of the pro-competitive strategy.

The question is: what lessons are to be drawn from this? Hibbard and Weeks (1989) continue:

> Decentralizing decision making and moving the locus of power from the provider to the consumer requires that the consumer is aware of this power shift and *is willing to exercise it*. Making this transition from patient to consumer may require stimulus [other] than simply financial incentives and access to information. It may call for more explicit cues and assistance in understanding this new role. That is, lack of information for health care choices may only be one part of the barrier in creating an active consumerate. (emphasis added)

Clearly, the strategy of trying to convert patients to consumers in the more market-orientated sense of the latter is one way of proceeding to influence the impact of patient payment on health care choices and thereby efficiency. And Hibbard and Weeks are surely right when they say that 'an active informed consumerate is the cornerstone of the pro-competitive strategy'. If they succeed in creating this 'active informed consumerate', then the pro-competitive strategy will surely work. But what if they cannot? Or if they cannot except at very high cost? Or if that is not what patients want? What then?

There is a need for more research here specifically on the question of the effects of knowledge of price – patient payment more precisely – on patient behaviour and health care utilisation.

It is worth pausing to appreciate that when we are discussing operational efficiency in health care we are talking principally about what doctors do and medical decision-making. In 1989, together with a medical colleague, Anne Loft, I edited a special issue of the *International Journal of Health Planning and Management* on the topic 'Best Medical Practice' (see Loft and Mooney, 1989). The point about this is not (necessarily) to encourage you to read the articles. Rather, it is to point out that the reason we set up the special issue was because there seemed no general agreement about how best medical practice should be defined conceptually. As it happens, several of the contributors (and not just the economists!) defined best medical practice as operationally efficient medical practice. Given that defining that in practice is so difficult, it is not surprising that it is difficult to come up with evidence of the effect of competition or any other form of incentive on operational efficiency. It is even more difficult to interpret what little evidence does exist!

Maybe yet again, as with effectiveness, the question is not so much one of the efficiency of hospitals but rather the efficiency of doctors. To say that, of course, does not mean that competition between hospitals will not change the behaviour of doctors. There does, however, seem to be a need within such a frame to study the effects of incentives on the individual doctors. One thing to note in considering the evidence on competition is that medical doctors in the United States are normally not a part of the hospital but operate independently. Their concern for the hospital and for its costs may thus be less than in other countries where the doctor's employment status *vis-à-vis* the hospital is very often different.

That brings us to allocative efficiency. Stoddart (1989) remarks in this context: 'as a tool for efficiency . . . incentives seem best suited to the lower-level objectives of technical efficiency, clinical appropriateness, and cost-effectiveness rather than allocative efficiency, where the complexity of the task increases as social evaluations of output must be made.' Competition could be a force in moulding resource allocation in response to social values – a task normally performed by the price mechanism in other markets. But it is difficult to see just how this might work in health care markets, unless of course (as is possible) the doctor-agents can reflect the social valuations. The question then would need to be: is competition the best way of achieving this? And that is where there have to be very serious doubts. It may be possible to set up a system of incentives to allow all of this to happen but it is not clear that the existence of competition is more likely to allow it to happen.

Equity? There seems little doubt that competition, whatever its other virtues, is not the way to provide incentives for the promotion of equity in health care.

The last item on the list above is change. It is here that the key element may lie. In the United Kingdom much of what is being sought could have been obtained within the existing structure and without the ideas of competition and contracting. The same is true, for example, of the reforms in the New Zealand health service. Given, however, the conservative nature of the British NHS, and health services more generally, one has to wonder whether the changes would have occurred (even if they *could* have occurred) without competition and contracting. It is probably an unanswerable question. I make the point, however, simply to emphasise that getting other changes through in health care may require a quite radical approach to the system if the parts are to be overhauled.

In a particularly useful paper on privatisation in Canada, Stoddart and Labelle (1985) suggest from their survey of the evidence that 'where efficiency improvement has been achieved, the determining factor has not been the degree of public versus private control, but rather the degree to which payment responsibility and decision-making authority are brought together to serve well-defined objectives of the enterprise.' Maynard (1982) comments in similar vein on the lack of ability of systems *per se* to solve the problems of efficiency. (More generally, for a review of the systems – public and private, inter-nationally – even if a little old now, see McLachlan and Maynard, 1982. For a more recent review of aspects on the financing side, see Donaldson and Gerard, 1993.)

It is difficult to reach any very definite or very general conclusions about competition and its merits. The evidence is rather thin and often rather specific to particular settings. Elements of competition and certain forms of competition may well be justified. Competition more generally in the more market-orientated form of neoclassical econ-omics seems unlikely to be an efficient basis for health care given the nature of the commodity and consumers' lack of information. Certain-ly, incentives need greater attention in most health care systems and it may well be that certain aspects of competition will figure among the most efficient forms of incentives.

Here again we can see that it is not possible to get efficiency in health care without efficient doctors. Patient payments are a less useful tool to promote such efficiency than is the remuneration system for doctors. The latter is likely to be better in policy. This preference stems largely from the fact that doctors have more influence over resource use than patients have. It is also partly a result of the lack of information that patients bring to their consumption decisions in health care. We know doctor remuneration systems 'work' in the sense that doctors do act differently to some extent at least under different systems. Where we need more information is on three fronts. First, we need to know more about what the objectives are that we as societies want from the health care system. Second, we need to know what efficient medical practice is. And third, we need more information than we currently have about precisely how different forms of remuneration, fee structures, etc., influence how the doctors practise. Then societies can hope to pursue the goals of health care efficiently, thereby maximising society's social welfare and at the same time allowing doctors to maximise their utility.

UK NHS reforms

I have already written at some length in *Economics, Medicine and Health Care* and in *Health Policy* (Donaldson and Mooney, 1993) about the NHS reforms *per se*. However, here I want to consider the issue of the purchaser/provider split, specifically in the context of this chapter, i.e. seen from the point of view of incentives.

The reforms have as a central tenet that competition is 'a good thing', although this is restricted to competition in provision and not in financing. Whereas purchasing and providing used to be done through the one body, now they are separate, with health authorities and GP budget holders doing the purchasing, and providers both in the public sector and the private sector 'competing' for business from the purchasers. GP fundholding means that general practices with a list size of at least 11,000 patients can purchase certain types of services directly on behalf of their patients. On the provider side, there are NHS trusts, which are managerially autonomous; directly managed units, which remain controlled by the health authorities directly; and facilities in the private sector.

Given this structure and some of the problems already identified above on the need for a number of firms in any market, for example, if competition is to be successful, there has to be some doubt about the prospects of this experiment working. As Shackley and Healey (1993) remark: 'Whether the benefits of competition will be realised in practice depends largely upon the prevalence of the necessary market conditions for a competitive provider environment.' Yet there are many parts of the United Kingdom where there will be little competition in the sense of several 'firms' competing for the business from the purchasers. Indeed, for some services (and sometimes many) in some parts of the country there will be a single provider.

Much will depend on the relative strengths of the two sides, and frequently it will be the case that a monopolist on one side will be faced with a monopsonist on the other. What the outcome will be is impossible to predict in principle. In practice, it will depend very much on how well each side bargains and uses the potential strength of their respective position. As Shackley and Healey (1993) stress: 'the outcome is in general indeterminate and crucially depends upon the relative bargaining strengths of the monopolist and the monopsonist.'

Where one might expect the market to work is where there is a situation with many providers competing within a relatively small area. London is clearly the place for that, but unfortunately from the point of view of seeing how this 'internal market' is working the market in London has, to all intents, been abandoned or at least suspended.

Despite these doubts about whether the soil is fertile for competition to work in the 'new' NHS, it is relevant to ask whether, when the circumstances are right, it can work. In the context of operational efficiency what would seem to be crucial is that there is some mechanism to ensure that quality is maintained and that purchasers are well placed to be able to judge on quality. Information on costs, or at least prices, will be clearly visible so that is less of a problem. However, the visibility of quality or effectiveness will be much less.

There is a sense in which this has been recognised, with the emphasis that is being placed on medical audit in the NHS at the present time. Indeed this aspect of the reforms would seem to be crucial. How successful this will be will be heavily dependent on how it is done and what incentives there will be to get the doctors to pay attention to what emerges from the audit studies. As indicated elsewhere in this book (see Chapter 8) there have to be doubts about the likely success of the efforts here unless there is more concern to relate medical audit more directly to operational efficiency and not just to effectiveness, as is currently the case. Designing 'Rolls Royce' medical practices without considering cost will lead only to frustration on the part of both doctors and health service administrators. In turn this may well eventually lead to the process of audit being discredited. Costs – that is, opportunity costs – need to be just as central in medical audit as benefits. There is little evidence that this is being recognised in the medical audit initiatives being pursued in the NHS reforms.

Additionally, there is a need to recognise that practice guidelines emerging from audit are not enough. Incentives to get medical practice and medical practitioners to change are needed. As indicated in Chapter 10, there is good evidence that doctors do respond differently to different forms of incentives. What is needed, yet again, is more evidence on what is efficient practice through an efficiency-based form of audit and then incentives put in place to get health services to deliver that efficient practice. This sort of strategy does not seem to be being put in place to support the operational efficiency goals of the 'internal market'. It may be here that the market will flounder.

On the allocative efficiency level, there are three aspects that would seem relevant in the reforms. First, will there be more explicit priority setting between different competing programmes such as those for the elderly or the mentally ill or for maternity care? If such priority setting is more conscious and explicit, it may also be more open and less determined (as in the past) by medical professional values and power. That in itself would make an important contribution to the possible achievement of better allocative efficiency. There would appear to be grounds for hope here. Second, given the thrust of the market mechanisms, it would seem likely that the priority accorded to acute care versus the traditional 'Cinderella' long-term care pro-grammes – geriatrics and psychiatry – will be enhanced in the future even more than in the past. This would not seem to reflect accurately the social values with respect to such care and as a result allocative efficiency may lose out here. However, there is a third aspect to this and that is the move towards attempting to establish 'community values' to support priority setting in the reformed NHS. If this is successful, then it may serve as a counter to the point just made. However, to date the work that has been done on trying to establish such values has seemed somewhat misdirected and one has to wonder to what extent this is little more than political gimmickry or simply part of the public relations exercise in selling the reforms to the British people.

There would, I believe, be general agreement that the internal market will do nothing to support the equity goals of the NHS and indeed is likely to work against these.

However, as indicated by Shackley and Healey (1993), we must wait to see how in the event the process works out. The success of the market in the NHS will in the end be a matter for empirical evidence rather than economic theorising – at least with respect to efficiency – even if we can express doubts about the likelihood of success. We must wait and see. However, a judgement – a negative one – can be made now with respect to equity.

What is still more difficult is to judge, even if the internal market does 'work', is whether there might not have been better ways of achieving such success. The evidence and the theorising would seem to suggest that there may well be better ways. These lie in deciding clearly what the objectives of health care are to be and what incentives are best suited to getting us there – especially our doctors. The kinds of incentive that competition provides may be a part of that ideal package of incentives. However, there seems no *a priori* reason to believe so.

Conclusion

Competition can, of course, take all sorts of forms. So too can incentive structures more generally. What the evidence suggests to date is that competition in health care is unlikely to be the best mechanism for providing the right incentives for efficiency or equity in health care. It may help with efficiency but is most unlikely to promote equity. The challenge for the modern health care systems is to find those sets of incentives which are appropriate to health care rather than rely on outmoded and inappropriate models of competition. What gives grounds for hope that this search will begin in earnest is the very fact that competition is seemingly so popular. Policy makers do want to pursue change to get better health services. The popularity of competition will wane quickly when it fails to deliver. Then the search for a better set of incentives will be pursued in earnest. Consequently, the current emphasis on competition is perhaps best seen as a necessary – if unfortunate – stepping-stone to creating the right incentive structures for the health services of the next century.

References

Andersen, T. F. and Mooney, G. H. (1990) *The Challenges of Medical Practice Variations*. Macmillan, London.

Culyer, A. J. and Posnett, J. (1990) Hospital behaviour and competition. In A. J. Culyer, A. Maynard and J. Posnett (eds), *Competition in Health Care, Reforming the NHS*. Macmillan, London.

Donaldson, C. and Gerard, K. (1993) *The Economics of Health Care Financing. The Visible Hand*. Macmillan, London.

Donaldson, C. and Mooney, G. (1993) The new NHS in a global context: is it taking us to where we want to be? *Health Policy*, **25**, 6–19.

Hibbard, J. H. and Weeks, E. C. (1989) Does the dissemination of comparative data on physician fees affect consumer use of services? *Medical Care*, **27**, 12, 1167–74.

Loewy, E. H. (1990) *Textbook of Medical Ethics*. Plenum, New York and London.

Loft, A. and Mooney, G. (1989) Special Issue on 'Best Medical Practice'. *International Journal of Health Planning and Management*, July/September.

McLachlan, G. and Maynard, A. (eds) (1982) *The Public/Private Mix for Health*. Nuffield Provincial Hospitals Trust, London.

Maynard, A. (1982) The regulation of the market. In G. McLachlan and A. Maynard (eds), *The Public/Private Mix for Health*. Nuffield Provincial Hospitals Trust, London.

Melnick, G. A. and Zwanziger, J. (1988) Hospital behaviour under competition and cost containment policies. *Journal of American Medical Association*, **260**, 2669–75.

Monroe, K. B. and Krishman, R. (1984) The effect of price on subjective product evaluation. In J. Jacoby and J. Olson (eds), *Consumers of Merchandise and Store Quality*. D. C. Heath, Lexington, Mass.

Mooney, G. (1992) *Economics, Medicine and Health Care*. 2nd edition. Harvester Wheatsheaf, Hemel Hempstead.

Rice, T. H. and Labelle, R. J. (1989) Do physicians induce demand for medical services? *Journal of Health Politics, Policy and Law*, 14, 587–600.

Sager, M. A., Easterling, D. V., Kindig, D. A. and Anderson, D. W. (1989) Changes in the location of death after passage of Medicare's prospective payment system. *New England Journal of Medicine*, 320, 433–9.

Shackley, P. and Healey, A. (1993) Creating a market: an economic analysis of the purchaser provider model, *Health Policy*, 25, 153–68.

Stoddart, G. L. (1989) Incentives for efficiency. Paper presented at the European Conference in Health Economics. Barcelona.

Stoddart, G. L., and Labelle, R. J. (1985) Privatization in the Canadian Health Care System. Discussion Paper, Policy, Planning and Information Branch, Health and Welfare, Canada.

11

What do we want from our health services? What can we expect from our doctors?

Introduction

There is a concluding chapter to this book. Originally though, I thought that this might be it. This chapter brings together quite a lot of the strands and issues that have been addressed. An earlier version of the paper was presented as the Distinguished Lecture in 1992 at CHEPA, McMaster University. I am grateful to my friends at CHEPA for allowing me to reproduce that paper here.

The chapter represents an attempt on my part to look at the state of health economics and of health services and to bring these together on two key issues. First, what do societies set as objectives for their health services? This is a matter that, for reasons that are not clear to this observer, does not get adequately addressed (although see Leeder, 1992). For example, in the reforms of the UK NHS there was much less attention given to the issue than might reasonably have been expected. One of the results of this has been that it is difficult to indicate the extent of 'success' of these reforms because there are no clear performance indicators. Again in the New Zealand reforms, while it is the case that, initially, there was deemed to be inequity of access to what ought to have been the same services across the country, in practice the extent to which this remains reflected in the operational objectives and indeed even the objectives in principle is no longer so clear. Second, what are doctors trying to do? Clearly, they are trying to treat their patients, but what does that mean in practice? What is the aim of that treatment? Are there other goals that doctors carry with them into the consulting rooms? Doctors do not neglect totally considerations other than the health or utility of their patients.

They do change their practice patterns for reasons other than the health status of the patient in front of them, and doctors faced with similar patients do treat them differently.

While much of what is in this chapter is health economics, its focus is very much policy. In developing the material for this chapter I took heart from a paper by Lomas (1991). In discussing the implications of his research for the development of practice guidelines, Lomas mentions three aspects, the last of which is that 'payers for and reviewers of medical care bemoan the lack of impact on clinical behaviour of practice guidelines.' This lack does seem to exist. Lomas' point, however, raises interesting questions about what the targets of the guidelines are – what do we want our doctors to do? – and whether guidelines are the best way of ensuring that the targets get hit. It is these issues *inter alia* that I want to address in this chapter.

The basic tenet on which the chapter is built is that central to the whole question of efficiency in health care is the efficiency of doctors. We cannot have efficient health services without efficient doctors.

The standard analysis of neoclassical economics with demand and supply being independent from one another and the informed consumer in the marketplace exercising his or her rights over his or her consumption decisions is at best a very poor description of what is happening in the health care market.

The nature of health care for the patient is such that the doctor frequently acts as a type of 'agent' to the ill-informed patient to assist the patient to maximise his or her health and/or his or her utility. Given such a role, the doctor is operating on both the demand and the supply side of the market. (This agency role is seen by economists as important in health care. It involves the better-informed doctor acting as an agent for and on behalf of the ill-informed patient.)

Yet the doctor, as the patient's agent, cannot easily perform all the tasks fully and in a wholly informed way on behalf of the patient. Only the patient can make the link, for example, between health status changes and changes in the patient's own utility.

But additionally, while there is a tendency for health care to be seen and analysed by economists primarily at the level of the individual patient or group of patients, it is necessary to recognise the concept of the institution of health services as something for which the citizenry has certain wishes. There is a need to consider the role of agency at this level too and perhaps to accept that the problems that exist here may be related to a failure by societies to establish better what the appropriate distribution of responsibility is with respect to health services decision making. In other words, who is to decide about what and at what level?

In the next section I shall consider in more detail the role of agency in health care. In the third section I will address the question: 'What do we want from our health care services?' Here my concern is not so much to answer the question but rather to suggest that economists have very seldom addressed it. Thereafter in the fourth section I will consider the issue: 'What can we expect from our doctors?', looking at the sorts of analyses that have been conducted by economists of doctors' behaviour but, more important, trying to examine a little what we know of the incentives facing doctors.

I will also suggest the sort of research agenda required to identify ways to get these agency roles to work better and the sorts of policy issue that are likely to be generated in addressing these matters.

Health care and agency

It is accepted by most health economists that the nature of the commodity health care is such that it cannot be exchanged efficiently in normal markets (Arrow, 1963; McGuire *et al.*, 1988). While there are a number of reasons for this, perhaps the issue of asymmetry of information is most crucial. Consumers (or patients) lack information to be able to make rational informed choices – they have at best imperfect knowledge of the nature of the health problem and the availability and effectiveness of treatments. Doctors are better informed. Yet they, the doctors, cannot make the final link between health status changes and changes in the utility of the patient. This link can only be made by the patient.

In this context the notion of agency (Evans, 1984) comes into play. The ill-informed patient has to rely, to some extent, on the better informed doctor for help. Two questions arise with respect to this statement of the agency role. To what extent do patients rely on their doctors? And what is it that the doctor is trying to achieve through helping the patient?

Despite the central role of agency in health economics, there is a lack of agreement among economists about what it is that the agent is trying to maximise. Williams (1988) has suggested, for example, that 'the "consumers" rely on doctors to act as their agents, in a system which ostensibly works on the principle that the doctor's role is to give the patient all the information the patient needs in order to enable the patient to make a decision, and the doctor should then implement that decision once the patient has made it.' Here the doctor is maximising patient information so that the patient can then make a rational informed decision. And given what he says elsewhere (Williams, 1985), it appears that the way for the patient to maximise his or her utility is through maximising solely health.

Culyer (1991) has a somewhat similar but importantly different view of agency. He describes the agency relationship as involving 'medical doctors, who act as agents on his or her (the patient's) behalf: ideally choosing in the way the individual would, had he or she been possessed of the same informational advantages of the professional'.

Here, note three things. First, the goal of agency is again information. Second, it is the doctor who does the choosing (and not, as with Williams, the patient). And third, the only apparent difference between what the doctor would choose and what the patient would choose is the different levels of information from which they start. The patient, having been informed by the doctor, would make the same decision as the doctor then makes. Again from his views elsewhere (Culyer, 1988, 1989) it seems that all Culyer allows to influence the patient's utility is health.

A third view of agency comes from Evans (1984). He seems more concerned with the maximisation of patient utility than with either patient information maximisation or patient health maximisation. Just what would be contained in patient utility beyond health Evans leaves somewhat unclear, but has expressed the view elsewhere that it is the patients' preferences that should determine this (Evans and Wolfson, 1980).

Thus three leading health economists fail to agree on what agency in health care is trying to maximise. Does this disagreement matter? That is for the reader to judge although my view would be that it does. I would tend to favour Evans' view of agency, essentially that what is to be maximised is the patient's utility and that what is contained in this should be determined by that patient's preferences. If we take Williams' or Culyer's view, concerns are restricted to health. Many doctors might well agree with that view of their agency role; however, such medicalisation of the patient's utility (and perhaps of health economics) is neither defensible nor desirable.

But there is a further important point to be made here with respect to Culyer's and Williams' views. In Williams' description of agency, the patient makes the decision after being informed by the agent. It has to be the case here then, if the goal is to maximise patient utility, that either the process of decision making in all cases generates positive utility or at least there is no loss of utility to the patient if the patient makes the decision. In Culyer's view, there is no potential for allowing positive utility in decision making by the patient. Further, there is no prospect or allowance for the possibility that the informed preferences of the patient will be different from the informed preferences of the doctor.

There is another agency issue here that merits mention, even if briefly, but which has been little investigated to date. For the individual as a citizen, he or she has certain 'wants' with respect to a health care system as a social institution which go beyond the concerns that that individual has in the role of a patient. (The most obvious here relates to equity.) The ill-informed citizen faced with uncertainty has to rely to some extent on a better informed politician or policy maker (the agent) to help in making choices. Precisely who embodies this agency role is not so clear; it is unlikely to be the doctor (although many doctors may be less clear about that).

It is important in this context to consider the values on which health care services as social institutions are based and how, for example, these values may vary from country to country. While the sources of such variations in values are likely to be several, one in particular is highly relevant to the theme of this chapter: the concept of autonomy. At a time when autonomy, at least in European health care services, is such an important and topical issue, I want to discuss later the different forms that autonomy might take. For the moment, I simply want to establish the notion of a citizen's agent for the health care system.

What do we want from our health care services?

Patients' utility

It would be understandable if, from the above, the reader were led to believe that it was for doctors to decide what factors affected patients' utility, both positively and negatively. But that cannot be acceptable. There has to be some way of finding out, and more scientifically than economists have attempted to do to date, what it is that patients want from their doctors. There is some limited evidence on this issue.

Let me exemplify from one area in particular. In prenatal screening there has been a tendency for economists in economic evaluations to assume that the only influence on the screened woman's utility relates to the opportunity to abort an affected foetus (although for an important exception here, see Feeny and Torrance, 1989). Yet it is clear that there are other potential sources of utility in such a screening programme.

Let me mention a few. For the screened population the information from the screen may be valuable either in itself or for reasons other than deciding to abort an affected foetus. This must surely be the case since, for some such screening tests, a substantial proportion of women screened positive do not abort (from various surveys about 16 per cent in Duchenne muscular dystrophy, and 41 per cent in haemophilia, Lubs and Falk, 1977; ' ıd for polycystic kidney disease about 50 per cent of women screened, Macnicol *et al.*, 1986).

Additionally, for those screened and informed that the foetus is not affected, there is the reassurance involved in gaining this knowledge.

For non-screened women, however, there is also the possibility of the screening programme having an impact on their utility. Here there are two groups who might be affected. First, there are those women who, though eligible, choose not to be screened and then regret later that they were not. Second, there are those who are deemed to be not eligible for screening. I have suggested elsewhere (Mooney and Lange, 1993) that this group may suffer 'deprivation disutility'. Whether a screening service exists or not, they are not screened, but when such a service does exist, they know of its existence and they know they are excluded. Then the argument is that being 'deprived' causes them loss of utility.

Such screening highlights the possibility of another influence on patients' utility. In the presence of a screening service, women are faced with various choices which do not exist in the absence of such a programme. These include whether to be screened and whether to abort if there is some problem with the foetus. If we concentrate solely on health status as the only influence on the utility of the women, then there is no prospect of including the loss of utility associated with making difficult decisions.

The point is not necessarily to argue for the inclusion of these particular influences on the patient's utility. Rather, it is to suggest that there may be influences beyond health that patients will want their agents to take into account. Indeed the questions of decision making and of information lead back to the earlier discussions in this paper with respect to the disagreement among economists about the nature of the agency relationship.

Patients may suffer utility gains or losses from making decisions; this will be true of information as well. If either or both of these statements is right, and if these are seen as legitimate concerns in considering patient utility, then that would provide support for the view that what the agent should be trying to maximise is patient utility and not information, as Williams suggests, or health, as Culyer suggests. But we need evidence. We have too little at present, largely because, as economists at least, we have seldom sought it.

Citizens' utility

It will be clear to the reader that what I have been addressing above relates mainly to what we might want from our physicians rather than what is the wider concern in the first question in my title: what do we want from our health care services? I now want to move out from the narrower patient perspective to the wider citizen perspective, which I raised briefly earlier in this chapter in the discussion on agency. While there may be various arguments that might be added at this level – and we might debate what these are – I simply want to suggest that there are additional arguments to be considered at this level; and second, there is a need to clarify these more than has occurred to date.

Let me exemplify that in the context of equity. Recently, there has been a debate running among health economists over the question of defining equity in health care (Wagstaff *et al.*, 1991; Mooney *et al.*, 1991; Culyer *et al.*, 1992a; Culyer *et al.*, 1992b; Mooney *et al.*, 1992). Culyer and his colleagues appear to be consequentialists in the sense that what, in their view, provides utility is only the consequences of acts. It is only states of the world that provide utility. I tend to think that there are other sources and that some of these may be most appropriately designated under the heading of 'process utility', or utility associated with doing or taking part.

Consequentialism in this context of equity pushes Culyer and his colleagues to argue that the equity goal in health care has to be health. I look first at what governments are saying and doing in this field, and second at what individuals appear to wish and, echoing Evans and Wolfson (1980), argue that what influences individuals' utility should be first determined by the individuals and second accepted by economists. It is not for us to judge the morality or simply goodness of one set of influences over another.

Taking all that into account, I end up supporting a definition of equity which is defined in terms of equal access. This is not consequentialism, however; it is some form of process; or following Margolis (1982) and his fair shares model, then it may be explainable in terms of a desire on the part of citizens simply to make health care services available to the whole society. Whether or not, having done so, they then use these services is not an issue.

Yet the great majority of research efforts of economists on equity have gone into measuring either inequalities in health or inequalities in use, consumption or expenditure. This to me is a process akin to that of weighing heat. We have a measuring rod. Then we look for a definition which suits our measuring rod. Since there is a weighing machine, let us find something we can weigh.

There can be little doubt that whatever the problems in measuring health and health care utilisation, they are less than those in measuring access which is even difficult to define. But rather than get on with defining access and finding a measure of access, health economists have tended to adopt what I think are inappropriate consequentialist notions. For me these are either wrongly based philosophically or are adopted simply because we can measure them.

Let me use the opportunity to quote from Nye Bevan, who was the architect of the UK NHS. In his vision of the NHS, Bevan wrote (see Foot, 1975): 'No society can legitimately call itself civilized if a sick person is denied medical aid because of lack of means.' And he continued, in one of my very favourite quotes: 'Society becomes more wholesome, more serene, and spiritually healthier, if it knows that its citizens have at the back of their consciousness the knowledge that not only themselves, but all their fellows, have access, when ill, to the best that medical skill can provide.'

Here I think we have evidence at a political level of the concern for equity in health care, a concern which is by no means unique to the UK health service and indeed falls well short of being fulfilled as an objective in that service. I think the question of the equity goal of health services is one that can influence the citizen's utility – as Bevan put it – the knowledge that all in society have access to care.

There may be other arguments at this level and there may be others like equity that need debate and clarification. There is not space to pursue them here and indeed all I want to establish is that there is scope for including, debating and clarifying additional arguments at this 'health services for the citizen' level as compared to the 'health care for the patient' level.

With respect to the citizen's utility, I mentioned earlier that autonomy may be rather important. I want to expand a little on this concept, as I think it is one which is in danger of being devalued and oversold currently in some health care systems (e.g. the United Kingdom). One might want to note in passing that to devalue and oversell a product at the same time requires a quite extraordinary set of skills. Or maybe it is simply that if a statement is made often enough – such as 'patient choice is a good thing' or 'an important goal of any caring health service is to give patients the opportunity to choose' – then enough people will choose to believe it.

With respect to the issue of choice and autonomy, let me say very firmly:

1. I am not aware of any empirical evidence that health care services with greater patient choice are generally more efficient than others; and
2. I am not aware of any empirical evidence that patients or citizens

generally want more choice rather than less choice. (Indeed in the United Kingdom, where the government has promoted this idea that choice *per se* enhances utility, I am not aware that patients or citizens have been asked if they want more choice. But maybe those peddling autonomy do not believe in giving people a choice over whether they want choice in their health care.)

Autonomy, as I have discovered in working with the Danish philosopher Uffe Juul Jensen, is a complicated concept. With his help, but with considerably less skill than he has, let me expose some of the intricacies involved (for more detail, see Jensen and Mooney, 1990).

There are three main forms of autonomy:

1. Deontological autonomy.
2. Relativistic autonomy.
3. Social autonomy.

The first of these, which I think is the most commonly found, suggests that the patient has the right to decide for himself or herself between various therapeutic strategies, or to decide if he or she wants treatment at all, or to use health care services at all.

Under deontological autonomy, we are free to act responsibly but without taking into account our personal inclinations and attitudes as individuals as to whether we want to act in this way. You will choose. Choice is good for you. Paternalism is belittling.

This is to be compared with the second form of autonomy – relativistic autonomy – in which each individual has a right to adopt his or her own preferences. The individual's own preferences should be taken into account. Here, as compared with deontological autonomy, the patient has the choice as to whether or not his or her preferences are counted.

This is much closer to my own view of what autonomy ought to be about, and the reader will immediately see that this allows me to incorporate, within the influences on individuals' utility, anything that the individual wants included, whether it is consequentialist or not.

The third form, social autonomy, implies a rejection of individualism (which is endorsed by both deontological autonomy and relativistic autonomy). Values are common – they are social values.

Rights and obligations are acquired in social contexts. They determine power and dependence between individuals. And this form of autonomy in turn leads to the notion of societies having a responsibility for the weak.

In laying out these different definitions of autonomy it is not my intent to argue the superiority of one over another. I am simply pointing to the fact that since there are different concepts of autonomy, there is a need to be clear what we mean by autonomy and to accept that autonomy itself is a value-based concept.

Does this question of autonomy matter? I think it does because it allows, *inter alia*, an explanation of why different societies organise their health care systems differently. Or in the language of this chapter, why we might expect that what the Canadian citizen wants from her health care services may well be different from what the Scot or the Dane wants from hers.

More fundamentally, I think we need some sort of effort at consistency in the values we bring to considerations of what we want from our health care services.

It is at this level, too, of the citizen's utility that the QALY league table would apply, assuming that it is to apply at any level. Now I would want to be very careful in making any criticism of what has been said in favour of such mechanisms for priority setting (for more detailed analysis of this issue, see Birch and Gafni, 1992; Gerard and Mooney, 1993). Work undertaken by Gerard (1992) on the quality and comparability of CUA studies indicates further that we need to be cautious in using QALY league tables. The specific point I would want to make in the context of this chapter however is the very simple one that QALY league tables assume that the only thing we want from our health care services is health.

In summary, what we want from our health care services is less than clear, but in my view includes important characteristics that extend beyond health (however that is defined). Contenders include information, reassurance, decision making, avoiding difficult decisions, avoiding regret, avoiding deprivation and the promotion of equity. I do not know if they are all there; I do not know how important they are *vis-à-vis* health. More worrying, I am convinced that I am not alone in my ignorance, at least not among my fellow health economists.

What can we expect from our doctors?

Having discussed at some length the issue of what we want from our health care services, let me be a little more concise in my comments with respect to doctors' abilities or capacities or desires to provide what we want.

Perhaps the best way forward in addressing this is simply to ask: why should we expect doctors to provide what we want? They may be trained in the delivery of health care or at least health care treatments but disagree, or at best be uncertain, as to how best to do that and even more so with respect to how to deliver health. They are little trained, if at all, in eliciting from patients what it is that influences patients' utility. It is far from clear that they see their agency role extending beyond the health arguments. With respect to these health arguments, it is not clear that they believe that what is best for their patients in health terms is to be determined on the basis of patients' preferences rather than their own (i.e. the doctors') preferences.

Given the complications I have introduced above with respect to the nature of what it is that we want from our health services, and given the inability of doctors to agree (as evidenced in the medical practice variations literature – see, for example, Ham, 1989) as to what is best even in simple health terms for their patients, can we really expect doctors to deliver in terms of what we want from our health care services?

Perhaps by asking about health care services in my first question and about doctors in my second, I could be accused of creating the prospect of a poorer 'match' than would have existed if I had stuck to doctors or health care services in both questions. However, in doing so, it was my intention to point to the fact that we cannot expect doctors to deliver what we want from our health care services, but that by altering their behaviour we can go a long way in getting the health care services to deliver what we want. In the end, in this respect, we have to rely on health care services and not on doctors.

In health care policy we need more often to act to influence doctors' behaviour. There has been a tendency, which somehow will not die, to assume that through the code of ethics with which doctors operate, they will somehow deliver what societies want from their doctors and from their health care services.

Now if this were the case, it would be difficult to believe that medical practice variations would be as great or take the form that they do. Yet there is substantial evidence to show that there are significant variations in medical practice for virtually all conditions where such variations have been mapped. In other words, left to their own devices doctors will largely 'do their own thing'. It is unlikely that all of them are practising efficient care; indeed, given the variations that exist, it seems at best that a small minority can be practising efficient care. However, we do not for most forms of treatment know what efficient care is. Additionally, while we might be confident that some doctors are practising efficiently, we don't know which ones.

More important still in this context, if there were some ethically correct doctor behaviour which they all practised, the nature of the remuneration and incentive structures facing doctors would not affect their behaviour. Yet they do.

This is not a cause for regret or dismay; indeed, it is a cause for rejoicing. As indicated in Chapter 9 (Krasnick *et al.*, 1990), the change in GP remuneration in Copenhagen from capitation to joint capitation/ FFS resulted in substantial changes in servicing of patients. Doctors can be influenced by how they are paid. Where, however, we have too little knowledge is with respect to just exactly what the impact of these incentives is on actual behaviour. We have an important policy tool, but our knowledge of its workings is grossly deficient.

It is also clear from the general economics literature on agency (see, for example, Arrow, 1986) that the nature of the optimal payment system to ensure that the agent (doctor) acts in the best interests of the patient is complex. To get the doctor to act as a perfect agent requires very sophisticated and well-researched remuneration systems for doctors, especially given what is written above about what it is that we want from our health services. Yet this is an area of health economics where we know so little.

What we can expect from our doctors is certainly not what we want from our health services. What we want is rather complex and we need much more research to determine what that is and in more detail than we have at present. But even if it were the case that we only wanted maximisation of health, then it is far from clear that the incentive structures are in place to allow such maximisation to occur. Given that we seem to be wanting more than just health, then the complexity of the agency role grows and with it the need to research much more deeply and much more appropriately into the nature of medical decision making and in particular what doctors want from the health care system.

If we are to get the incentives right to get agency to work efficiently, we need to know what we are trying to achieve. We need to investigate thoroughly what we want from our health care services and then devise the incentives to provide the means to get there.

The lack of research and sophistication surrounding physician incentives is worrying, and I am puzzled that economists seem so relatively silent on the issue. As economists we are in a position to research into incentives, perhaps better than just about any other discipline. Yet economists and others are so ignorant of how to get our doctors to deliver what society wants them to deliver. We cannot expect them to deliver what we want them to deliver, when what we want is so unclear.

Yet somehow this seems to be what we do expect, or at least the lack of research on this topic implies either that we do or that the issue is not important in research or policy terms. I cannot believe that.

I am convinced that to get our objectives for health care clearly and explicitly stated matters and that then devising a structure of incentives to get our health care services, and especially our doctors, to get us there, ought to be the central issue in health services research and the research of health economists, at the present time. What we want from our health care services, we simply cannot rationally expect our doctors to deliver. I would submit that it is time our research, the research of health economists, of policy analysts and of health services researchers generally, reflected that fact.

References

Arrow, K. J. (1963) Uncertainty and the welfare economics of medical care. *American Economic Review*, **53**, 941–73.

Arrow, K. J. (1986) Agency and the market. In K. J. Arrow and M. D. Intrilligator (eds), *Handbook of Mathematical Economics*, vol. III. Elsevier, Amsterdam.

Birch, S. and Gafni, A. (1992) Cost effectiveness/utility analyses: do current decision rules lead us to where we want to be? *Journal of Health Economics*, **11**, 279–96.

Culyer, A. J. (1988) Inequality of health services is, in general, desirable. In D. Green (ed.), *Acceptable Inequalities?* Institute of Economic Affairs, London.

Culyer, A. J. (1989) The normative economics of health care finance and provision. *Oxford Review of Economic Policy*, **5**, 34–58.

Culyer, A. J. (1991) Competition and markets in health care: what we know and what we don't. NHS White Paper, Occasional paper No. 3, Centre for Health Economics, York.

Culyer, A. J., van Doorslaer, E. and Wagstaff, A. (1992a) Comment. Utilisation as a measure of equity by Mooney, Hall, Donaldson and Gerard. *Journal of Health Economics*, **11**, 93–8.

Culyer, A., van Doorslaer, E. and Wagstaff, A. (1992b) Access, utilisation and equity: a further comment. *Journal of Health Economics*, **11**, 207–10.

Evans, R. G. (1984) *Strained Mercy: The economics of Canadian health care.* Butterworth, Toronto.

Evans, R. G. and Wolfson, A. D. (1980) Faith, hope and charity: health care in the utility function. Discussion paper 80–46, Department of Economics, University of British Columbia, Vancouver.

Feeny, D. and Torrance, G. W. (1989) Incorporating utility-based quality of life assessment measures in clinical trials: two examples. *Medical Care*, March, S/190–204.

Foot, M. (1975) *Aneurin Bevan, 1945–1960*. Paladin, London.

Gerard, K. (1992) Cost-utility in practice: a policy maker's guide to the state of the art. *Health Policy*, **21**, 249–79.

Gerard, K. and Mooney, G. (1993) QALY league tables; handle with care. *Health Economics*, **2**, 59–64.

Ham, C. (1989) *Health Care Variations: Assessing the evidence.* The King's Fund Institute, London.

Jensen, U. J. and Mooney, G. H. (1990) *Changing Values in Medical and Health Care Decision Making.* Wiley, London.

Krasnick, A. *et al.* (1990) Changing remuneration systems: effects on activity in general practice. *British Medical Journal*, **300**, 1698–701.

Leeder, S. R. (1992) Valuable health: what do we want and how do we get it? Sidney Sax Oration. *Australian Journal of Public Health*, **16**, 6–14.

Lomas, J. (1991) Making clinical policy explicit: legislative policy-making and lessons for practice guideline development. Working paper 91–12, McMaster University Centre for Health Economics and Policy Analysis, Hamilton.

Lubs, M. L. and Falk, R. F. (1977) Response of relatives to prospective genetic counselling in severe X-linked disorders. In M. L. Lubs and F. de La Cruz (eds), *Genetic Counselling.* Raven Press, New York.

Macnicol, A. M., Watson, M. L. and Wright, A. F. (1986) Implications of a genetic screening programme for polycystic kidney disease. *Aspects of Renal Care*, **1**, 219–22.

Margolis, H. (1982) *Selfishness, Altruism and Rationality.* Cambridge University Press, Cambridge.

McGuire, A., Henderson, J. and Mooney, G. (1988) *The Economics of Health Care.* Routledge and Kegan Paul, London.

Mooney, G. H. and Lange, M. (1993) Ante-natal screening: what constitutes benefit? *Social Science and Medicine*, **37**, 7, 873–8.

Mooney, G., Hall, J., Donaldson, C. and Gerard, K. (1991) Utilisation as a measure of equity: weighing heat? *Journal of Health Economics*, **10**, 475–80.

Mooney, G., Hall, J., Donaldson, C. and Gerard, K. (1992) Reweighing heat: response to Culyer, van Doorslaer and Wagstaff. *Journal of Health Economics*, **11**, 199–205.

Wagstaff, A., van Doorslaer, E. and Paci, P. (1991) On the measurement of horizontal inequity in the delivery of health care. *Journal of Health Economics*, **10**, 169–206.

Williams, A. (1985) Economics of coronary artery bypass grafting. *British Medical Journal*, **291**, 326–9.

Williams, A. (1988) Priority setting in public and private health care: a guide through the methodological jungle. *Journal of Health Economics*, **7**, 173–83.

12
Where now with health economics?

Introduction

In this chapter I want to consider why it is that there seems relatively little use made of economics generally in health care policy making. I trust that that will not make the chapter sound like special pleading on behalf of health economics. I also hope that readers will accept that it is legitimate to discuss such a matter at the end of a book which has attempted to show that economics does have a contribution to make, at least at the level of principles, to health care issues and in a number of different ways.

The next section looks at the results from three surveys that have been done in Australia, Denmark and the United Kingdom to examine the questions of why economics is not being used more in health care and what might be done to improve the position.

Thereafter, drawing on this and also on other experiences, I have tried to come up with some explicit suggestions as to how best health services can get a better return from health economics and make better and more use of health economists.

Some evidence from three countries

The Australian evidence

This was compiled by Jayne Ross in her MPH thesis at the University of Sydney (Ross, 1992). Her survey was of decision makers at both the

Commonwealth (federal) level and the state (in this case, New South Wales) health departments and relates purely but usefully to economic evaluation, not to economics more generally.

With respect to the constraints on greater use of economic evaluation, Ross concluded:

> The main barrier to the use of economic evaluation identified by the decision makers was in relation to its practicality in the decision-making environment within which they operated. They perceived that it took too long in an environment where decisions have to be made quickly. That the decision-making process also had to take into account existing policy and political factors as well as other issues was seen as a barrier to using economic evaluation.

She identified the other main barriers as 'communication between health economists and decision makers, clinical imperatives, availability of data and appropriate management systems and lack of knowledge and expertise in economic evaluation'.

The policy implications that flow from these barriers to use, if that use is to be improved, are fairly obvious, but Ross highlights one in particular: 'Those advocating or conducting economic evaluations need to be responsive to the decision makers' needs.' She adds that it is important that the analysts have a better grasp of the decision environment they are trying to influence. She also highlights the need for education in economic evaluation but counsels against too great an emphasis on this, in essence because of the opportunity cost involved. In other words, there are very few health economists around to do the studies and if they spend too much of their time on education, they will not be able to do the studies!

The Danish evidence

In Denmark, in 1988, a somewhat similar exercise was conducted by Marlene Gyldemark-Jorgensen (see Enemark *et al.*, 1990) based on a postal questionnaire sent to senior health service staff in different disciplines – medical doctors, nurses, administrators and politicians. In this case, however, the survey related to economic analysis more generally and not just economic appraisal.

According to those surveyed, the main reasons why economic analysis was not used more in the Danish health service were related primarily to lack of knowledge of economic analysis, misconceptions of economics and the fact that few people had the skills to conduct such analyses. Decision making was also seen as being 'too political' to allow economic analysis to have much influence.

In terms of possible solutions to these problems, education and training of staff in economic analysis figured prominently. There was also a strong view that there needed to be someone in the health services who would be identified as having responsibility for ensuring that economic analyses were carried out.

The UK evidence

The UK investigation was based on discussions at a workshop on Economic Appraisal in the NHS organised by the Health Economics Research Unit at the University of Aberdeen in early October 1983. (Clearly that is some time ago and things have moved on. However, no similar exercise has been conducted since but many of the issues remain as then. Where not, I have tried to indicate this.)

Participants at the workshop were senior health service staff and health ministry staff who already had some understanding of what economics is and what it is capable of doing (and not doing!). A report on the workshop is available (Ludbrook and Mooney, 1984).

The main problems identified in preventing the wider and better use of economic appraisal in the United Kingdom were as follows. First, there was a lack of awareness of economic appraisal, what it is and what can be expected of it. While things have improved over time, I would judge that this is still true today. Second, one of the most interesting aspects of the discussions at the workshop was that many participants recognised the single-mindedness with which clinicians pursue their patients' interests, that there was considerable agreement – and indeed sympathy – for this stand, and that there were few problems here. The fact that 'clinical freedom' is not recognised as a problem may, in practice, be one of the biggest hindrances to getting economic appraisal used.

Third, there were misconceptions about economic appraisal at a number of levels, but particularly with respect to the fact that economic appraisal studies were seen to be necessarily very time consuming and complex. Yet others felt they were really very simple; there was little to learn and economic appraisal was already widely practised.

Because many health services decisions are inevitably political, there was felt to be little point in performing economic appraisal studies. Further, the nature of the decision-making process is such that it was consequently difficult to introduce rational tools of analysis and difficult to identify precisely where the responsibility lay for doing so. Other problems related to resistance to new ideas and problems in applying economic appraisal, particularly lack of skills in the health service to do the studies, lack of clear objectives to be appraised, poor data and lack of availability of data. Interestingly, few participants saw problems with the methodology. Finally, participants expressed the view quite strongly that economists were poor at communicating with health service professionals.

Recommendations for attempting to overcome these problems were identified at three levels.

Under educational activities, the key areas identified were that top management should be seen as the target group for gaining acceptance of economic appraisal; that health economists should develop teaching packages which are genuinely pertinent to the needs of staff in the health service; that training in economic appraisal should formally include 'learning by doing'; and that 'crash courses' in health economics for NHS staff who already have degrees in economics should be organised.

Second, there were recommendations on initiatives for co-operation. The key issues here related to support of those in the service who were already interested to apply health economics. Particularly important here was the idea of creating the right decision-making framework in which efficiency and economic appraisal might flourish.

Third, there were ideas on how to provide more direct support for appraisal. These were fairly practical but the need for economists to improve their communication skills and their understanding of the health service decision-making environment were stressed.

Some assessment

There are some common messages emerging from these three studies. If we looked at other countries, somewhat similar lessons and ideas would almost certainly emerge. What I conclude from this is, first and foremost, that unless there is a demand for health economics there is no way that the thinking and techniques of health economics will take off to a greater extent than at present. There may be a need to alter the product in certain ways to make the product more acceptable and appealing to the potential consumers. It may be that it should be marketed better, for example, by more education drives to make the potential consumers more aware of the potential benefits that consumption would bestow. There are clearly various ways of stimulating demand.

Most fundamentally, however, as with any product, unless there is a market for it, it is a waste of resources to produce it. There have to be people who want the product. If there are not, then no amount of manipulation of the market will be successful in selling the product.

Too few health service personnel today want health economics. It is the explanation for that that seems to lie at the heart of any problem here.

Economics will only be used to any great extent in health care when efficiency becomes a key, day-to-day objective of health care services. As has been spelt out in various places in this book, the average doctor frequently has little incentive to try to pursue efficiency, and indeed it will more frequently be the case that it will be in the interests of both his or her patients and his or her own interests not to pursue efficiency. Given the importance of doctors in resource allocation decision making in health care, if they are not efficient, then efficiency will not be achieved. If they do not have an interest in pursuing efficiency, then they will not be interested in the use of economics in health care. Patients, although less influential in resource allocation in health care than consumers are in other markets, none the less also have little incentive as patients to pursue efficiency in health care. Indeed, those who do have an interest in efficiency – the managers, possibly, and the taxpayers or premium payers almost certainly – are often too far removed to be able to influence the efficiency of the system to any great extent. Managers and administrators often see their role as being one of oiling the system on behalf of the doctors rather than having goals which are separate from the doctors. Tax and premium payers are too often too far from decision making on health services and are confused about any distinction between their roles as patients and their roles as payers.

The lead has to come from the top, especially from politicians prepared to be answerable to their electorate for the sensible stewardship of health care funds and not to the emotionalism that so often surrounds health care decision making at the political level. Senior health service managers have a role here too. There is also a need to make health service management a much more attractive career than it currently is, with the relevant incentives to attract the very best managers. They have a horrendously difficult task. Yet in terms of financial rewards, job satisfaction and status, they come very far behind the health care professionals, especially the doctors, who in the end they are supposed to control. There is a need for fundamental change at that level.

What is somewhat depressing is the poor quality of much of the strategic decision making that emanates from health ministries and departments. In Chapter 3 I pointed to the weaknesses in the thinking present in such a strategic policy document as *The Health of the Nation* from the Department of Health. In the production of that document, there was an opportunity to promote good approaches to priority setting and to get the English health service moving in a sensible direction and at a time when, with the reforms the NHS faces, there was a cry for help from the service. It was missed. Other countries seem to fare little better. In Denmark there is an obsession with process, and the National Board for Health, which ought to be taking the lead in influencing how the health service in the counties is organised and planned, is failing to take the opportunity to promote good practice in terms of health service policy setting and instead promulgates clinical guidelines in the forlorn hope that these will in themselves influence the health services in Denmark to be more effective. Little or nothing is done at that level to promote efficiency.

In Australia, at the federal level, there are some grounds for hope with the sort of initiative that has been taken on the pharmaceuticals front, where it is now necessary to have an economic appraisal conducted before a product can be marketed. Why restrict such an edict to pharmaceuticals? But it is a start. At the level of priority setting in New South Wales, there is too great a similarity with *The Health of the Nation* approach and a risk that that document has become something of a trendsetter.

Trendsetting in health care policy making is an important phenomenon. One only has to look at the way that diagnosis-related groups (DRGs) have taken off across the world to see how there is a transferability of such policy technology from one country to another. Unfortunately – and DRGs are a case in point – the extent to which such transferability is done on an informed, rational basis seems more limited than one would ideally wish. It is possible to learn from others, but it is also important to understand properly why a particular approach was adopted in the place of origin. Then there is a need to see whether the local circumstances elsewhere merit the transfer of the approach to that place, and if so to what extent some sorts of adjustment are needed in doing so.

DRGing in health services is an international industry and with seemingly too little thought being given in countries outside the United States, where it originated, as to whether the problems these other countries face are sufficiently similar to those faced by the United States to justify transferring this particular technology. There is too little assessment as to whether DRGing has 'worked' in the United States in any sense that one would want to transfer it. Additionally, there is too little thought given to whether, even if it would work in other countries, there are not still better ways of promoting the same ends in these other countries.

Equity seems to fare little better, largely it appears because decision makers at the top levels mouth slogans but fail to deliver at an operational level. That would seem to be what is about to happen in New Zealand, where an overly strong equity goal which cannot be delivered is likely to result in substantial problems in delivering any more reasonable policy on equity at all.

I am sure there will be similar examples of problems at top policy levels in other countries; I can write only about those countries where I have most knowledge. The examples from these, however, do not suggest that at the top levels of health care decision making – whether political or bureaucratic – the opportunities that are there to promote more efficient and equitable health services are being taken.

It is consequently at this level that the product of efficiency needs to be sold and thereafter economics will follow. That means in turn that there needs to be much more debate about what societies want from their health services – what are the objectives of health care and is efficiency sufficiently high on that agenda to justify a major shift in the way that health services are organised, how doctors are trained and in what and how incentives can be structured to pursue these objectives? Then health economics will take off.

Health economists are very definitely also at fault. We could certainly do better at selling our wares. We are often poor communicators and we frequently fail to do enough market research to understand what the problems are that our product might actually be used to address in the market and how best to package the product to make it user friendly. Too often we sit on the sidelines wondering why we are ignored when we have not sought to answer the question and get involved in the game ourselves.

There are clear indications, as have been voiced at various stages of this book, that doctors are inefficient. At the same time, I have been at pains to point out that normally this is not their fault. They need to face the right sorts of incentive to get them to be efficient. Normally they do not. As economists, we need to try much more to understand the nature of medical decision making if we are to get these incentives right. Only when we understand why doctors behave as they do will we be well placed to decide how best to structure incentives to change that behaviour to promote efficiency. This is an area where there is scope for much better research by economists. At present the literature on medical decision-making by economists is at best crude in the way that it tries to model the doctor's utility function. (For a critique of this literature, see Kristiansen, 1993.)

Thus while we await the time – and I think the position is changing for the better in a number of countries – when health economics will be in much greater demand, one of the key areas for health economics research is medical decision making. Oddly, it has been relatively neglected by economists in the past. We need a much better understanding of doctors' behaviour, what incentives they currently face and how best to alter incentives to get doctors to behave more efficiently than they do at present.

There may not be a brave new world ahead for health economics. Yet with preparation now on these fronts, at least health economics will be better placed to respond to the demands of health services for increased efficiency if or when the call comes.

References

Enemark, U., Gullov, O., Lange, M. and Mooney, G. H. (1990) *Economic Evaluation and Priority Setting in Health Care.* Egmont Fonden, Copenhagen.

Kristiansen, I. S. (1993) What is in the doctor's utility function? Working paper, Institute for Social Medicine, University of Tromsø, Tromsø.

Ludbrook, A. and Mooney, G. (1984) *Economic Appraisal in the NHS. Problems and Challenges.* University of Aberdeen, Aberdeen.

Ross, J. (1992) Economic evaluation in health service decision making. MPH thesis, Department of Public Health, University of Sydney, Sydney.

Author index

Subject index

ability to pay, 74
access, definitions of, 81
adverse selection, 139
agency, 79, 87–103, 134, 139, 169,
    170–2
    and the citizen, 172
APKD (autosomal polycystic kidney
    disease), 17, 18
audit, 110
autonomy, 18, 19, 72, 159
    and choice, 175
    and decision making, 18–20
    deontological, 19, 176
    relativistic, 20, 176
    social, 176

baseline comparisons, 53
benefits, non-health, 55–6, 172–3
Bevan, Nye, 83
Black Report, 70
breast cancer, 45

capitation versus FFS, 126–35
CEA versus CUA, 61
changing health care, 162
choice
    and autonomy, 175
    and efficiency, 174–5
    and utility, 93
    freedom of, 100
clinical trials, 110
commodity, nature of the, 138

community values, 14, 15
competition, 152–63
    and agency, 99
    and equity, 152–3, 161
compliance, 78
consequentialism, 20, 174
consumer information, 142
consumerism, 160
consumer sovereignty, 19
co-payment, 74, 135–46
Copenhagen GP study, 126–35
cost–benefit analysis, 13
    of illness, 45–7
    reductions, 145
    utility analysis, 13
cost-effectiveness analysis; see CEA
cost-utility analysis, see CUA
cream skimming, 139
CUA studies, local, 58, 60–1, 63
    transferability, 58–9
CUA versus CEA, 61

demand and use, 106
    non-induced, 104–7
    supplier induced, 104–12, 131
deontological autonomy, 19, 176
deprivation disutility, 22
distributive justice, 66
Down's syndrome, 17, 18, 22
DRGs (diagnosis-related groups),
    109, 156–7, 187
drug evaluation, 62